COPD - Pathology, Diagnosis and Treatment, Consequences, and Future Directions

Edited by Steven A. Jones

Published in London, United Kingdom

COPD - Pathology, Diagnosis and Treatment, Consequences, and Future Directions
http://dx.doi.org/10.5772/intechopen.1001502
Edited by Steven A. Jones

Contributors
Abebe Ayalew Bekel, Abu Talha Hanfi, Adekunle M. Mofolorunso, Alexandre Semionov, Biruk Getahun, Bojan Kovacina, Dagnachew Zemene, Dessalegn Demeke Ayalew, Erstu Legese Beyene, Gideon Olamilekan Oluwatunase, Jasmina Biscevic-Tokic, Josephine Pressacco, Karl Sayegh, Khalid A. Ansari, Melkamu Demewez Gebeye, Nedim Tokic, Olayinka Olawale Asafa, Onome Bright Ogenetega, Oyovwi Mega Obukohwo, Patrick Godwin Okwute, Qurat Ul Ain, Samuel Olalekan, Sana Ahmad, Sanja Brekalo-Lazarevic, Steven A. Jones, Subba Digumarthy, Tahzeem Riaz, Yasha Sajjad, Zurifa Ajanovic

First published in London, United Kingdom, 2024 by IntechOpen
IntechOpen is the global imprint of INTECHOPEN LIMITED, registered in England and Wales, registration number: 11086078, 167-169 Great Portland Street, London, W1W 5PF, United Kingdom

British Library Cataloguing-in-Publication Data
A catalogue record for this book is available from the British Library

Additional hard and PDF copies can be obtained from orders@intechopen.com

COPD - Pathology, Diagnosis and Treatment, Consequences, and Future Directions
Edited by Steven A. Jones
p. cm.
Print ISBN 978-0-85466-344-6
Online ISBN 978-0-85466-343-9
eBook (PDF) ISBN 978-0-85466-345-3

For EU product safety concerns:
IN TECH d.o.o., Prolaz Marije Krucifikse Kozulić 3, 51000 Rijeka, Croatia,
info@intechopen.com or visit our website at intechopen.com.

Meet the editor

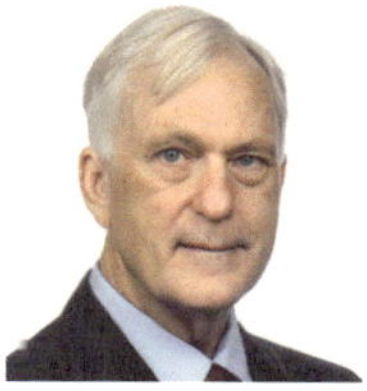

Dr. Jones received BA, MS, and Ph.D. degrees at the University of California, San Diego, with a focus on Bioengineering and Fluid Mechanics and Signal Analysis. He was a Postdoctoral Fellow at the Georgia Institute of Technology and a Research Associate at Johns Hopkins, and is now the Wayne and Juanita Spinks Associate Professor of Biomedical Engineering at Louisiana Tech University. His area of interest is the application of fluid mechanics, mass transport, and feedback control (both positive and negative) to biomedical problems. He recently became interested in the problem of chronic obstructive pulmonary disease as one caring for someone with the pathology at the end stage, and he recognized that his engineering interests were strongly applicable to the disease. In that connection, he became interested in the underlying pathology of the disease, the conventional treatment options, and future directions in the understanding and treatment of the disease.

Contents

Preface

The rule of threes states that one can survive for three weeks without food, three days without water, but only three minutes without oxygen [1]. Consequently, anything that threatens the ability to take in oxygen is uncomfortable and potentially life-threatening. Chronic obstructive pulmonary disease (COPD) does so through multiple mechanisms, including an increase in the effort required to ventilate the lung alveoli, lost alveolar elasticity, restricted bronchi, and inefficient transfer of oxygen to the blood.

While the risk of lung cancer from smoking is well known by the general population, the risk of COPD is less familiar, except for patients with the disease or their families and caretakers. Even people familiar with the acronym COPD may not be able to describe the disease physiologically. Nonetheless, the mortality burden of the disease is high, and COPD is variously reported as the third or fourth leading cause of death [2]. It may be less important to state the exact ranking than to note that the disease has a mortality similar to that of stroke and Alzheimer's disease [3, 4]. The ranking in undeveloped countries, where wood burning for cooking and work-related chemical exposure is more prevalent, tends to be higher than that in developed countries, where the primary cause is smoking.

Having been the primary caretaker for a family member (Flo) with end-stage COPD, I was excited to have the opportunity to edit this book. Flo's experience informs some of the details highlighted within this book. She was a life-long smoker who had been diagnosed with COPD, but initially, her COPD was not debilitating. In 2020 she contracted a severe case of COVID-19 that led her to the intensive care unit for a week. Afterward, her COPD had advanced to the extent that she was placed in hospice. Ultimately, after about a year of hospice, she had a fall and broke her hip. Although the hip was repaired, it became difficult to carry through with the rehabilitation process, and that, along with repeated infections, led to her death in January 2022.

The hospice nurses were knowledgeable and personable, but they could not answer certain of my questions because, as I later discovered, no definitive answer was available. Paramount among these questions was the mechanism through which a restoration of oxygen to the normal resting 96 to 99 percent in COPD patients led to hypercapnia. This situation was frustrating for me as a biomedical engineer, and it made me realize that many of the subject areas in which I had expertise were directly applicable to the search for answers to some of these questions—specifically, airway and blood flow relate to fluid mechanics, gas exchange in the alveoli relates to mass transport, and the processes of inflammation, respiratory drive, and remodeling relate to feedback control. Thus, my reasons for editing this book are both personal and professional.

Several themes are repeated throughout this book. The first is the question of why, as a society, we need to confront COPD. An objective reason is the cost that the disease adds to healthcare and to the loss in productivity of patients and caretakers. The more important reason is the suffering that the individual patients must endure from the disease. As both health professionals and humans, we have an instinct that drives us to help those who are suffering.

A second theme is the multifaceted nature of the disease. The criterion for diagnosis of COPD is simplistic, stated as a ratio of forced expiratory volume in one second to forced vital capacity less than 70%, as measured with spirometry. However, the underlying mechanisms for the decrease in this ratio vary from patient to patient. The primary mechanisms are bronchitis, affecting the bronchi, and emphysema, affecting the alveoli. Patients may have one or the other, or they may be affected to different extents by both. Furthermore, bronchitis can have varying pathologies from patient to patient, where in one case the narrowing of the bronchi is dominant while in another case it is mucus formation. Similarly, emphysema can have varying degrees of alveolar surface area loss, elasticity loss, or other factors. Thus, while spirometry allows the physician to assign a name to the patient's condition, the diagnosis is not specific.

A third theme is the most frustrating one for COPD patients and physicians. The consensus is that COPD is a degenerative disease. Whereas the symptoms can be treated over the short term, no treatment is available to reverse the effects of COPD. Current therapies either slow the progression of the disease or help the patient to live with the problem.

A fourth theme is that COPD itself is only part of the problem for these patients. The inability to adequately oxygenate tissues leads to other problems that are not strictly pulmonary in nature. With inadequate oxygenation, exercise becomes difficult, and as the disease progresses, even normal daily tasks become onerous. The consequent lack of motion causes atrophy of the muscles, including those involved in breathing, which in turn causes daily ac-tivities to be more difficult. As the body adapts to ineffective ventilation, the chest wall and diaphragm become altered such that they function less efficiently. Thus, COPD tends to worsen itself by mechanisms that are separate from the deterioration of lung tissue. Furthermore, the loss of muscle mass, and possibly other mechanisms, can affect the patient's balance and gait, leading to a higher likelihood of a fall that could lead to a broken bone, such as a hip. Recovery from such a break invariably relies on rehabilitation, which muscle degradation and chronic fatigue cause to be particularly difficult.

While conventional wisdom is that COPD cannot be cured or even reversed, several potential therapies have been investigated that have not yet been introduced in practice. These strategies are reviewed by Guarnier et al. [5], who also elucidate the multitude of basic science questions that must be answered before their practical application. Nonetheless, some success has been obtained in animal models through the use of stem cells [6, 7].

This book is composed of eight chapters. The introductory chapter, "Mathematical Modeling as Part of a Collaborative Effort to Improve COPD Treatment", emphasizes the need for future cross-disciplinary collaborations to make significant progress in the treatment of the disease. It is written from the point of view of a biomedical engineer. The second chapter, "The Complex Interplay: Unfolding the Mechanisms of Chronic Obstructive Pulmonary Disease", introduces the disease and emphasizes the complexity of its origins and mechanisms. The next two chap-ters discuss methods for COPD diagnosis and treatment. "Diagnosis and Management of Chronic Obstructive Pulmonary Disease" does so from a general perspective, and "Imaging of Emphysema: A Comprehensive Review" describes the manifestations on X-ray and other imaging modalities and provides guidance on separating different physiological aspects. The next three chapters discuss some consequences of the disease that might not be initially obvious. The fifith chapter, "Influence of Chronic Obstructive Pulmonary Disease on Work Ability", details the practical consequences of COPD on the ability to maintain employment and remain productive. The sixth and seventh chapter relate to the secondary effects of the disease, both of which are related to the critical risk of a disabling fall. "Balance Impairments in COPD" relates to the ability to maintain a stable posture, while "Chronic Obstructive Pulmonary Disease and Gait Disturbance: Is There Any Meaningful Link? Unveiling the Interplay and Addressing the Challenges" relates more specifically to ambulation. The final chapter, "Recent Advances in Chronic Obstructive Pulmonary Disease", addresses current research in COPD.

Steven A. Jones
Biomedical Engineering,
Louisiana Tech University,
Ruston, Louisiana, USA

References

[1] Towell C. Essential Survival Skills. London, New York: DK; 2011. 176 p

[2] Chen S, Kuhn M, Prettner K, Yu F, Yang T, Bärnighausen T, et al. The global economic burden of chronic obstructive pulmonary disease for 204 countries and territories in 2020-50: A health-augmented macroeconomic modelling study. Lancet Glob Health. Aug 2023;**11**(8):e1183-93

[3] Wu Y, Gao S, Zhou Y, Du C, Yang R. Trends in population mortality rates in the United States from 1969 to 2017. Annals of Palliative Medicine. Oct 2021;**10**(10):11035-11052

[4] Rana JS, Khan SS, Lloyd-Jones DM, Sidney S. Changes in mortality in top 10 causes of death from 2011 to 2018. Journal of General Internal Medicine. Aug 2021;**36**(8):2517-2518

[5] Guarnier LP, Moro LG, Lívero FA dos R, Faria CA de, Azevedo MF, Roma BP, et al. Regenerative and translational medicine in COPD: Hype and hope. European Respiratory Review. 30 Sep 2023

[6] Katsha AM, Ohkouchi S, Xin H, Kanehira M, Sun R, Nukiwa T, et al. Paracrine factors of multipotent stromal cells ameliorate lung injury in an elastase-induced emphysema model. Molecular Therapy. Jan 2011;**19**(1):196-203

[7] Huh JW, Kim SY, Lee JH, Lee JS, Van Ta Q, Kim M, et al. Bone marrow cells repair cigarette smoke-induced emphysema in rats. American Journal of Physiology-Lung Cellular and Molecular Physiology. Sep 2011;**301**(3):L255-266

Section 1

Introduction

Chapter 1

Introductory Chapter: Mathematical Modeling as Part of a Collaborative Effort to Improve COPD Treatment

Steven A. Jones

The current state of COPD treatment, in particular the inability to do much more than ease symptoms and slow the progression of the disease [1], underscores the need for extensive research into the condition and development of new strategies. This need cannot be fulfilled through a single discipline, but will require collaboration in fields of pathology, anatomy, genetics, engineering, physics, biochemistry, cell biology, informatics, microbiology, material science, clinical medicine, and numerous other areas. These fields have already contributed substantially to the current state of the art, and all continue to develop and use modern tools to continue their investigations. The relevance of mathematical modeling as a component in the development of new strategies may not be obvious to the general public, but modeling is supported by and supports more directly biologically related components. It is likely to be an important area of study as researchers investigate treatments that can not only halt progression of COPD but also reverse the disease's course.

Models are only as valid as the data that support them. They, along with the overall future directions in COPD therapy, will benefit from a greater understanding of fundamental pulmonary physiology and the complex interactions that occur among the gases, tissues, blood, antigens, pathways, genetic transcription, membrane permeabilities, and reaction kinetics. Biological and biochemical studies provide a wealth of information about the individual components of this physiology. Mathematical models can quantify these components to identify subtle changes in, for example, concentrations that may lead to substantial changes, therapeutic or pathological.

Multiple basic mechanisms remain unexplained related to both gas exchange and inflammation despite excellent relevant work that spans back over decades. It may not be surprising that the mechanism for matching perfusion with ventilation is unclear [2], given that the mechanism through which hypoxia increases blood flow in the peripheral circulation, a well-known and long-studied effect, is also unknown. Still, elucidation of the mechanism may have clinical applications. Similarly, the mechanism for hyperoxic hypercapnia is unknown, despite multiple studies and hypotheses [3, 4]. This phenomenon describes the increase in blood CO_2 that occurs when COPD patients are given supplementary oxygen that raises their resting blood oxygen saturation to the 96 to 99% levels that are considered normal. To avoid hypercapnia, physicians generally recommend that patients' saturation be kept between 88 and 92% [5].

The tendency for COPD to lead to worse COPD raises another pervasive theme, which is one of the positive feedback mechanisms in the disease. Some of these mechanisms are beneficial, such as the matching of blood flow with airflow. The matching can be considered as positive feedback because it implies that increased blood flow leads to increased airflow which in turn further increases blood flow. Of course, the effect is ultimately limited in normal physiology. COPD appears to disrupt this mechanism [6], leading to poor matching between ventilation and perfusion. Positive feedback is also present in the monocyte recruitment and macrophage activation processes of normal inflammation [7–10]. In contrast, COPD can trigger pathological positive feedback mechanisms, such as chronic inflammation that cannot resolve itself.

1. Clinical importance of modeling

Mathematical models can add to the overall understanding of pulmonary physiology. Because the behavior of the lung depends on excitatory and inhibitory pathways that interact with one another, the overall result of a change in chemical concentration, cellular mobility, timing delays, transport barriers, receptor densities, and other parameters can be unpredictable through qualitative analysis. It seems obvious that a regional increase in, for example, a vasodilator will lead to increased blood flow, but paradoxical effects can arise if the increase triggers a pathway that counteracts the effect. A good quantitative model can reveal these types of effects and can indicate which pathways are responsible for them. In vivo whole-animal models can similarly reveal these integrated phenomena but do not provide as much data. In instances where the model does not match the in vivo behavior, the discrepancy can be used to improve estimates of the time delays, production rates, receptor densities, and other parameters involved, and it may demonstrate the presence of a currently undiscovered component of the system. Thus, one fundamental role of modeling is to identify mathematical discrepancies in our current understanding of pulmonary physiology and to suggest additional experiments that should be done. The results of those experiments, combined with the consequent revised models, can suggest new potential clinical targets for treatment.

2. Systems that can be modeled

No model can describe a biological organ completely. To do so would require the model to account for every cell, cellular function, chemical agent, receptor, agonist, and subsystem in the organ and adjacent organs. COPD models therefore address specific aspects of the disease and pulmonary physiology. These aspects include flow in the airways, blood flow regulation, gas exchange, tissue remodeling, neural control, inflammation, mechanical stress, infection, and clearing of debris.

2.1 Airflow

Flow in the airways must consider the forces for inspiration and expiration, mainly those caused by the diaphragm and the intercostal muscles, the configuration of the lung lobes and the branching patterns of the airways, smooth muscle tone, mucus thickness, mucus viscosity, hydrostatic pressure, the elasticity of alveoli, bronchi, and bronchioles, and concentrations of oxygen, carbon dioxide, and nitric oxide. The models can, in theory, be specific to a given patient, but the vast amount of data that would be necessary to model a specific lung and the consequent computational requirements would be prohibitory. Thus, models tend to rely on general descriptions of a generic lung.

Specific rules are devised to describe the relationships between parent and daughter airways at branching locations. Much of our current understanding of this branching network comes from the meticulous studies of Weibel [11–13]. Islam et al. [14] reviewed models of the pulmonary airway tree and emphasized the importance of geometric configuration to both airflow and particle deposition. These models can help predict the amount of each gas species that enters the alveoli, the regions of the lung that are more susceptible to deposition of inflammatory particles, and optimal particle size for aerosol treatments.

For COPD, it is important to know how airflow is distributed to different regions of the lung. This distribution changes when airways become obstructed with mucus and narrowed by inflammation. In addition, the effort required for the patient to exhale increases as the alveoli lose elasticity. The increased pressure required to expel gas from the alveoli compresses the bronchi, tending to further narrow them and increase the difficulty of exhalation [15]. The patient compensates for this effect through the use of pursed-lip breathing, where the mouth is used to apply a back pressure on the airways to keep them open [16]. These mechanical issues have been reviewed by Bhana and Magan [17]. The ability of the alveoli to take in and expel gas, and hence the distribution of alveolar ventilation, is also affected by the surfactant. Ventzislava et al. demonstrated that the bronchoalveolar lavage fluid from COPD subjects had less surfactant lipids and proteins than that from non-COPD subjects [18]. Albert [19] proposed that when mechanical ventilation is used, it can decrease surfactant levels, which in turn increases damage to the alveoli.

2.2 Blood flow

Blood flow is the second half of the fluid mechanical aspects of lung function. As in airflow, blood flow occurs at length scales that vary over three orders of magnitude, and the considerations that arise at the length scales of the pulmonary artery and vein differ from those at the alveolar capillary level. Of particular importance is the regulation of blood flow to the arterioles and capillaries, as this determines the ability of the lung to match blood perfusion with alveolar ventilation [20]. Blood flow modeling at the arteriolar level requires not only that mechanical flow resistance be considered, but that the feedback mechanisms among shear stress, release of vasodilators and vasoconstrictors, endothelial and epithelial function, smooth muscle cell physiology, blood oxygen saturation, and transport barriers be considered [21–24].

2.3 Feedback/neural control

Neural control of breath rate and airflow volume is intriguing because it occurs both consciously and unconsciously. It is interesting from an engineering standpoint as both a feedback control problem and a transport problem that involves blood pH and blood concentrations of CO_2 and O_2. Although CO_2 is the primary driver of blood pH, chemoreceptors sense the two parameters separately [25]. An early model was published by Grodins et al. [26]. The component of respiratory drive that is governed by CO_2 arises from both peripheral chemoreceptors at the carotid bodies and a medullary chemoreceptor [15]. The carotid bodies also sense O_2. Overall, the neural respiratory drive is increased in patients with COPD [27] and the respiratory discomfort that these patients endure can arise from both excess CO_2 and from insufficient O_2.

Neural feedback control of pulmonary gas exchange is further complicated because the blood gas concentrations also affect pulmonary blood flow resistance, heart rate, cardiac output, and other parameters. Because the feedback mechanisms are both positive and negative [28], the effect of a single parameter becomes difficult to predict without a mathematical model that looks quantitatively at the complete system.

2.4 Gas exchange

Gas exchange is the most fundamental aspect of lung function. A quantitative study of gas exchange involves gas concentrations in the alveoli and blood, the transport barrier between the alveoli and the capillaries, the transport barrier between blood plasma and hemoglobin in the red blood cell, capillary blood flow, airflow, the kinetics of the interaction between O_2 and hemoglobin, the reactions involved in transport of CO_2 by plasma and the red blood cell, and the role of vasodilators such as nitric oxide in the control of both airflow and blood flow. One fundamental aspect of the interaction of CO_2 and O_2 with hemoglobin is the Bohr effect, which tends to offload more oxygen in a high CO_2 environment [29, 30] and the Haldane effect, which tends to offload more CO_2 in an oxygen-rich environment [29, 31].

Because overall gas exchange depends on blood flow and airflow, which in turn depend on neuronal control, studies tend to combine these effects into an integrated model [24]. Such models have been presented by Ursino's group at the University of Bologna [23, 32, 33] and by Tehrani [34]. These studies did not incorporate the effects of nitric oxide in their models. Buess et al. [35] specifically modeled the exchange of nitric oxide in the airways. They focused less on the vascular side of the pulmonary system, but rather considered blood to be a sink for nitric oxide.

2.5 Tissue remodeling

The ultimate treatment for COPD is to have the lung repair itself, which could mean the ambitious goal of reconstructing lost alveoli, or the more modest, but still ambitious goal of restoring the alveolar elasticity [36]. This therapeutic strategy requires an understanding of lung tissue remodeling that far exceeds current knowledge. It is known that lung tissue can remodel itself, but the remodeling can be pathological as much as therapeutic. Some insights can be gained from the changes in lung structure following lung reduction surgery, a procedure used in cases of severe hyperinflation [37]. In lung volume reduction surgery, a portion of the lung is removed to reduce lung volume, thus allowing the diaphragm and chest wall to operate at a volume that is more efficient [38].

Guarniere et al. [39] reviewed recent advances in the use of mesenchymal stem cells to promote tissue regenerating for COPD patients. They identified several major questions that must be answered before a viable method can be applied clinically. Among these are the cell culture environment and number of passages for the donor cells, cell dose, timing of the dose, route of administration, target tissue microenvironment, and localization of the cells to the target tissue (homing). Furthermore, the ability of mesenchymal stem cells to differentiate depends in a complicated manner on the chemical environment within the host. For example, while TGF-β promotes stem cell differentiation into smooth muscle cells [40], it also promotes the differentiation of epithelial cells to a mesenchymal phenotype [41]. This growth factor is one of the host of agents that must be present in the correct amount at the correct location to have the desired effect. These considerations illustrate how modeling of mass transport issues can support and in turn be supported by both in vivo and in vitro studies.

2.6 Inflammation

Chronic and recurrent inflammation is a hallmark of COPD [42] that leads to increased difficulty in breathing through production of excessive mucus [43] and to tissue damage [8]. Inflammatory cells, such as macrophages and lymphocytes, produce proteases [44] that promote degradation of alveolar connective tissue and cellular apoptosis [45]. Inflammation is initiated by triggers such as cigarette smoking, but it can persist years after smoking cessation [46]. Smoking appears to induce a change from an inflammatory process that is self-limiting to one that is self-perpetuating [42]. Such irreversible changes are characteristic of the branching solutions of nonlinear equations that can help to elucidate the underlying inflammation-perpetuating mechanisms.

2.7 Mechanical stress

Mechanical stresses are important to lung physiology on large and small scales, ranging from the muscular effort involved in respiration, to the elastic properties of the parenchyma that are relevant to ventilation efficiency [17], to the forces of mechanical ventilation that can lead to tissue damage [10, 47], and to the forces that lead to functional [48] and phenotypic changes in the numerous involved cell types [49]. The mechanical environment also affects the cycle of inflammation [49].

2.8 Infection

COPD exacerbations are particularly problematic in terms of morbidity, mortality, quality of life, COPD progression, and health care costs [50, 51]. Approximately half of all exacerbations are caused by infections, while irritants, allergic reactions, and other inflammatory triggers are also involved [50]. Common viral infections include rhinoviruses, influenza, parainfluenza, coronavirus, and adenovirus. Infections have been addressed mathematically in the case of acute respiratory distress syndrome [52].

Moxnes and Hausken [53] describe a viral infection model that describes the subsequent immune response. They compare the infections of H1N1 to H3N2 and noted a higher viral load and duration for the former. Dobrovolny et al. [54] reviewed eight mathematical models of influenza and compared quantifiable results to patient outcomes. Specifically, they examined those models where the authors had disabled cytotoxic T lymphocytes, antibodies, of interferon. None of the models were able to match all experiments, and the authors emphasized that additional work was needed both experimentally, to determine the important input parameters, and mathematically, to capture all important pathways.

2.9 Clearing of debris

Another aspect of pulmonary physiology that is relevant to COPD is the clearing of particulates from the airways. Mathematical models of this function were reviewed by Xu and Jiang [55]. The models must consider properties of the mucus (viscosity and viscoelasticity), the motion and coordination of the cilia, and additional forces such as those exerted by coughing.

3. Further questions to address

Several major questions need to be answered before significant progress can be made in treating, arresting, or reversing COPD. Some of these questions are clinical and require new methods to evaluate individual patients, map, and quantify regions of emphysema and bronchitis, characterize individual immune response, localize dead space, and quantify the spatial distributions of air and blood flow. With such measurements, it may be possible to treat each patient in a manner that is optimized to the individual's physiology. Other questions relate more to the specific mechanisms by which respiratory physiology adapts over short and long time spans.

3.1 Ventilation/perfusion matching

The mechanism through which the lung matches ventilation with blood perfusion is intriguing from the scientific standpoint in that it appears to operate in the opposite direction from the vascular control in the peripheral circulation. There, hypoxia increases blood flow, whereas in the lung, hypoxia decreases blood flow. The difference may result from a yet unidentified agent in the lung or it may be a result of phenotypic differences in the vascular cells (endothelial and smooth muscle) or an effect of the epithelial cells. More studies on the behavior of these cells, alone and in co-culture, may be helpful.

3.2 Hyperoxic hypercapnia

A general guideline for COPD patients on supplemental oxygen is to maintain oxygen saturation between 88 and 92% to avoid the tendency for hypercapnia that increases mortality risk [5, 56]. A better understanding of the mechanism by which high oxygen saturation leads to excess carbon dioxide in COPD patients might allow these patients to enjoy fully saturated blood without the dangers of hypercarbia. Multiple mechanisms have been suggested [4]. A computational study by Hanson et al. [57] suggests that the increase in dead space, coupled with the Haldane effect, is sufficient to explain this phenomenon. This conclusion is consistent with clinical measurements by Sassoon et al. [58]. It suggests that hyperoxic hypercapnia should vary with a patient's specific COPD physiology (e.g., degree of dead space) and that the 88–92% rule may not be appropriate for all COPD patients.

3.3 Inflammation and exacerbation

A third major question relates to the mechanisms through which inflammation is perpetuated even after smoking cessation and the causes of inflammation-induced exacerbations. While it seems intuitive that exacerbations must be triggered by an external stimulus, rates of exacerbations and their time courses vary from patient to patient [50], and variations in immune responses are likely responsible for some of this variability. A detailed analysis of an individual's immune response may help to predict the time course of an exacerbation and inform treatment. It is well known that positive feedback systems can lead to oscillatory behaviors [59], and given that inflammation includes positive feedback aspects, it is reasonable to propose that some episodes of exacerbation are not immediately triggered events, but are the consequence of a natural, though pathological, cycle in certain COPD patients.

3.4 Remodeling

Promotion of lung tissue remodeling through stem cell therapy, tissue engineering, genetic engineering, or other manipulations of cell growth and differentiation is a goal that is probably years from being reached. Achievement of this goal will require meticulous mechanistic experiments on the molecular, cellular, and tissue level. The problem thus lends itself to multiscale modeling [60] and can benefit from advancements in those techniques.

4. Conclusion

Further advancements in the treatment of COPD will require a concerted effort by researchers from a wide variety of fields. The associated problems are challenging, but well worth addressing for the health, well-being, and quality of life of the patients. Mathematical modeling can contribute significantly to an understanding of the mechanisms involved in COPD and to the development of modern treatments of the disease.

Author details

Steven A. Jones
Louisiana Tech University, USA

*Address all correspondence to: sajones@latech.edu

References

[1] Vogelmeier CF, Román-Rodríguez M, Singh D, Han MK, Rodríguez-Roisin R, Ferguson GT. Goals of COPD treatment: Focus on symptoms and exacerbations. Respiratory Medicine. 2020;**166**:105938. DOI: 10.1016/j.rmed.2020.105938

[2] Nagaraj C et al. Hypoxic vascular response and ventilation/perfusion matching in end-stage COPD may depend on p22phox. European Respiratory Journal. 2017;**50**(1):1601651. DOI: 10.1183/13993003.01651-2016

[3] Abdo WF, Heunks LM. Oxygen-induced hypercapnia in COPD: Myths and facts. Critical Care. 2012;**16**(5):323. DOI: 10.1186/cc11475

[4] Sarkar M, Madabhavi I, Kadakol N. Oxygen-induced hypercapnia: Physiological mechanisms and clinical implications. Monaldi Archives for Chest Disease. 18 Nov 2022;**93**(3):101-113

[5] Echevarria C, Steer J, Wason J, Bourke S. Oxygen therapy and inpatient mortality in COPD exacerbation. Emergency Medicine Journal. 2021;**38**(3):170-177. DOI: 10.1136/emermed-2019-209257

[6] Neder JA et al. V/Q mismatch: A novel target for COPD treatment. Chest. 2022;**162**(5):1030-1047. DOI: 10.1016/j.chest.2022.03.033

[7] Ceresa M, Olivares A, Noailly J, González Ballester M. Coupled immunological and biomechanical model of emphysema progression - PMC. Frontiers in Physiology. 2018;**9**:1-16

[8] Brown BN et al. An agent-based model of inflammation and fibrosis following particulate exposure in the lung. Mathematical Biosciences. 2011;**231**(2):186-196. DOI: 10.1016/j.mbs.2011.03.005

[9] Cooper RL. An Applied Mathematics Approach to Modeling Inflammation: Hematopoietic Bone Marrow Stem Cells, Systemic Estrogen and Wound Healing and Gas Exchange in the Lungs and Body. Ph.D. Dissertation, Virginia Commonwealth University; 2015.

[10] Minucci SB, Heise RL, Reynolds AM. Review of mathematical modeling of the inflammatory response in lung infections and injuries. Frontiers in Applied Mathematics and Statistics. 2020;**6**:1-25. Available from: https://www.frontiersin.org/articles/10.3389/fams.2020.00036 [Accessed: February 7, 2024]

[11] Weibel ER. Morphometry of the Human Lung. New York: Springer Verlag and Academic Press; 1963

[12] Hsia CCW. Quantitative morphology of compensatory lung growth. European Respiratory Review. 2006;**15**(101):148-156. DOI: 10.1183/09059180.00010105

[13] Hsia CCW, Hyde DM, Weibel ER. Lung structure and the intrinsic challenges of gas exchange. Comprehensive Physiology. 2016;**6**(2):827-895. DOI: 10.1002/cphy.c150028

[14] Islam MS, Paul G, Ong HX, Young PM, Gu YT, Saha SC. A review of respiratory anatomical development, air flow characterization and particle deposition. International Journal of Environmental Research and Public Health. 2020;**17**(2):Art. no. 2. DOI: 10.3390/ijerph17020380

[15] Ferguson GT. Why does the lung hyperinflate? Proceedings of

the American Thoracic Society. 2006;**3**(2):176-179. DOI: 10.1513/pats.200508-094DO

[16] Yawn BP, Mintz ML, Doherty DE. GOLD in practice: Chronic obstructive pulmonary disease treatment and Management in the Primary Care Setting. International Journal of Chronic Obstructive Pulmonary Disease. 2021;**16**:289-299. DOI: 10.2147/COPD.S222664

[17] Bhana RH, Magan AB. Lung mechanics: A review of solid mechanical elasticity in lung parenchyma. Journal of Elasticity. 2023;**153**(1):53-117. DOI: 10.1007/s10659-022-09973-6

[18] Hristova VA et al. Multiomics links global surfactant dysregulation with airflow obstruction and emphysema in COPD. ERJ Open Research. 2023;**9**(3):1-17. DOI: 10.1183/23120541.00378-2022

[19] Albert RK. The role of ventilation-induced surfactant dysfunction and atelectasis in causing acute respiratory distress syndrome. American Journal of Respiratory and Critical Care Medicine. 2012;**185**(7):702-708. DOI: 10.1164/rccm.201109-1667PP

[20] Marquis AD, Beard DA, Finsky DJ. Towards a multi-scale model of ventilation-perfusion matching. The FASEB Journal. 2019;**33**(S1):lb455-lb455. DOI: 10.1096/fasebj.2019.33.1_supplement.lb455

[21] Jacob M, Chappell D, Becker BF. Regulation of blood flow and volume exchange across the microcirculation. Critical Care. 2016;**20**(1):319. DOI: 10.1186/s13054-016-1485-0

[22] Tawhai MH, Burrowes KS. Modelling pulmonary blood flow. Respiratory Physiology & Neurobiology. 2008;**163**(1-3):150-157. DOI: 10.1016/j.resp.2008.02.016

[23] Ursino M, Magosso E. Acute cardiovascular response to isocapnic hypoxia. I. A mathematical model. American Journal of Physiology-Heart and Circulatory Physiology. 2000;**279**(1):H149-H165. DOI: 10.1152/ajpheart.2000.279.1.H149

[24] Ursino M, Magosso E. Acute cardiovascular response to isocapnic hypoxia. II. Model validation. American Journal of Physiology. Heart and Circulatory Physiology. 2000;**279**(1):H166-H175. DOI: 10.1152/ajpheart.2000.279.1.H166

[25] Yoon S, Zuccarello M, Rapoport RM. pCO2 and pH regulation of cerebral blood flow. Frontiers in Physiology. 2012;**3**:365. DOI: 10.3389/fphys.2012.00365

[26] Grodins FS, Buell J, Bart AJ. Mathematical analysis and digital simulation of the respiratory control system. Journal of Applied Physiology. 1967;**22**(2):260-276

[27] Jolley CJ, Moxham J. A physiological model of patient-reported breathlessness during daily activities in COPD. European Respiratory Review. 2009;**18**(112):66-79. DOI: 10.1183/09059180.00000809

[28] Sylvester JT, Shimoda LA, Aaronson PI, Ward JPT. Hypoxic pulmonary vasoconstriction. Physiological Reviews. 2012;**92**(1):367-520. DOI: 10.1152/physrev.00041.2010

[29] Malte H, Lykkeboe G. The Bohr/Haldane effect: A model-based uncovering of the full extent of its impact on O 2 delivery to and CO 2 removal from tissues. Journal of Applied

Physiology. 2018;**125**(3):916-922. DOI: 10.1152/japplphysiol.00140.2018

[30] Malte H, Lykkeboe G, Wang T. The magnitude of the Bohr effect profoundly influences the shape and position of the blood oxygen equilibrium curve. Comparative Biochemistry and Physiology Part A: Molecular & Integrative Physiology. 2021;**254**:110880. DOI: 10.1016/j.cbpa.2020.110880

[31] Teboul J-L, Scheeren T. Understanding the Haldane effect. Intensive Care Medicine. 2017;**43**(1):91-93. DOI: 10.1007/s00134-016-4261-3

[32] Albanese A, Cheng L, Ursino M, Chbat NW. An Integrated Mathematical Model of the Human Cardiopulmonary System: Model Development. American Journal of Physiology-Heart and Circulatory 310: H899 –H921, 2016

[33] Albanese A, Chbat NW, Ursino M. Transient respiratory response to hypercapnia: Analysis via a cardiopulmonary simulation model. 2011 Annual International Conference of the IEEE Engineering in Medicine and 2011 Annual International Conference of the IEEE Engineering in Medicine and Biology Society. 2011. pp. 2395-2398.

[34] Moxnes JF, Hausken K. Mathematical modelling of acute virus influenza a infections. Mathematical and Computer Modelling of Dynamical Systems. 2012;**18**(5):521-528

[35] Buess A, Van Muylem A, Nonclercq A, Haut B. Modeling of the transport and exchange of a gas species in lungs with an asymmetric branching pattern. Application to nitric oxide. Frontiers in Physiology. 2020:570015. Available from: https://www.frontiersin.org/article/10.3389/fphys.2020.570015;**11**:570015. [Accessed: June 9, 2022]

[36] Río Bocos C, Jahn AK, Martin Medina A, Calvo Bota AM, De Francisco Casado MT, Pont Antona PJ, et al. Mesenchymal Stem Cells from COPD Patients Are Capable of Restoring Elastase-Induced Emphysema in a Murine Experimental Model. International Journal of Molecular Sciences. 15 Nov 2023;**24**:1-15

[37] Caviezel C et al. Identification of target zones for lung volume reduction surgery using three-dimensional computed tomography rendering. ERJ Open Research. 2020;**6**(3):00305-02020. DOI: 10.1183/23120541.00305-2020

[38] Gordon M, Duffy S, Criner GJ. Lung volume reduction surgery or bronchoscopic lung volume reduction: Is there an algorithm for allocation? Journal of Thoracic Disease. 2018;**10**(Suppl 23):S2816-S2823. DOI: 10.21037/jtd.2018.05.118

[39] Guarnier LP et al. Regenerative and translational medicine in COPD: Hype and hope. European Respiratory Review. 2023;**32**(169):220223. DOI: 10.1183/16000617.0223-2022

[40] Wang M-K, Sun H-Q, Xiang Y-C, Jiang F, Su Y-P, Zou Z-M. Different roles of TGF-β in the multi-lineage differentiation of stem cells. World Journal of Stem Cells. 2012;**4**(5):28-34. DOI: 10.4252/wjsc.v4.i5.28

[41] He H et al. Medicine targeting epithelial-mesenchymal transition to treat airway remodeling and pulmonary fibrosis progression. Canadian Respiratory Journal. 2023;**2023**:e3291957. DOI: 10.1155/2023/3291957

[42] Oudijk E-JD, Lammers J-WJ, Koenderman L. Systemic inflammation

in chronic obstructive pulmonary disease. European Respiratory Journal. 2003;**22**(46 suppl):5s-13s. DOI: 10.1183/09031936.03.00004603a

[43] Brightling C, Greening N. Airway inflammation in COPD: Progress to precision medicine. European Respiratory Journal. 2019;**54**(2):1900651. DOI: 10.1183/13993003.00651-2019

[44] Chakraborty K, Bhattacharyya A. Role of proteases in inflammatory lung diseases - PMC. Advances in Biochemistry in Health and Disease. 2013;7:361-385

[45] Barnes PJ. The cytokine network in chronic obstructive pulmonary disease. American Journal of Respiratory Cell and Molecular Biology. 2009;**41**(6):631-638. DOI: 10.1165/rcmb.2009-0220TR

[46] Willemse BWM, Postma DS, Timens W, ten Hacken NHT. The impact of smoking cessation on respiratory symptoms, lung function, airway hyperresponsiveness and inflammation. European Respiratory Journal. 2004;**23**(3):464-476. DOI: 10.1183/09031936.04.00012704

[47] Weaver L et al. High risk of patient self-inflicted lung injury in COVID-19 with frequently encountered spontaneous breathing patterns: A computational modelling study. Annals of Intensive Care. 2021;**11**:1-8. DOI: 10.1186/s13613-021-00904-7

[48] Andrabi SM et al. Nitric oxide: Physiological functions, delivery, and biomedical applications. Advanced Science. 2023;**10**(30):2303259. DOI: 10.1002/advs.202303259

[49] Hill MR et al. A theoretical model of inflammation- and mechanotransduction-driven asthmatic airway remodelling. Biomechanics and Modeling in Mechanobiology. 2018;**17**(5):1451-1470. DOI: 10.1007/s10237-018-1037-4

[50] Wedzicha JA, Donaldson GC. Exacerbations of chronic obstructive pulmonary disease. Respiratory Care. 2003;**48**(12):1204-1215

[51] Papi A, Luppi F, Franco F, Fabbri LM. Pathophysiology of exacerbations of chronic obstructive pulmonary disease. Proceedings of the American Thoracic Society. 2006;**3**(3):245-251. DOI: 10.1513/pats.200512-125SF

[52] McCahon RA, Columb MO, Mahajan RP, Hardman JG. Validation and application of a high-fidelity, computational model of acute respiratory distress syndrome to the examination of the indices of oxygenation at constant lung-state. British Journal of Anaesthesia. 2008;**101**(3):358-365. DOI: 10.1093/bja/aen181

[53] Moxnes JF, Hausken K. Mathematical modelling of acute virus influenza a infections. Mathematical and Computer Modelling of Dynamical Systems, 2012;**18**(5):521-528

[54] Dobrovolny HM, Reddy MB, Kamal MA, Rayner CR, Beauchemin CAA. Assessing mathematical models of influenza infections using features of the immune response. PLoS One. 2013;**8**(2):e57088. DOI: 10.1371/journal.pone.0057088

[55] Xu L, Jiang Y. Mathematical modeling of Mucociliary clearance: A mini-review. Cells. 2019;**8**(7):Art. no. 7. DOI: 10.3390/cells8070736

[56] Csoma B et al. Hypercapnia in COPD: Causes, consequences, and therapy. Journal of Clinical Medicine. 2022;**11**(11):Art. no. 11. DOI: 10.3390/jcm11113180

[57] Hanson CW, Marshall BE, Frasch HF, Marshall C. Causes of hypercarbia with oxygen therapy in patients with chronic obstructive pulmonary disease. Critical Care Medicine. 1996;**24**(1):23-28. DOI: 10.1097/00003246-199601000-00007

[58] Sassoon CSH, Hassell KT, Mahutte CK. Hyperoxic-induced hypercapnia in stable chronic obstructive pulmonary disease. The American Review of Respiratory Disease. 1987;**135**(4):907-911. DOI: 10.1164/arrd.1987.135.4.907

[59] Kundu PK, Chatterjee S. Nonlinear feedback self-excitation of modal oscillations in a class of under-actuated two degrees-of-freedom mechanical systems. International Journal of Non-Linear Mechanics. 2021;**135**:103768. DOI: 10.1016/j.ijnonlinmec.2021.103768

[60] Fletcher AG, Osborne JM. Seven challenges in the multiscale modeling of multicellular tissues. WIREs Mechanisms of Disease. 2022;**14**(1):e1527. DOI: 10.1002/wsbm.1527

Section 2

Pathology

Chapter 2

The Complex Interplay: Unfolding the Mechanisms of Chronic Obstructive Pulmonary Disease

Patrick Godwin Okwute, Adekunle M. Mofolorunso, Gideon Olamilekan Oluwatunase, Olayinka Olawale Asafa, Samuel Olalekan, Onome Bright Ogenetega and Oyovwi Mega Obukohwo

Abstract

Chronic obstructive pulmonary disease (COPD) is a widely prevalent respiratory ailment that can be prevented. It is characterized by the chronic restriction of airflow caused by lung abnormalities resulting from exposure to toxic chemicals or particles. COPD is a respiratory disorder characterized by a gradual and incapacitating progression, impacting a significant number of individuals on a global scale. COPD is distinguished by the presence of chronic bronchitis and emphysema, resulting in considerable morbidity and mortality. The etiology of COPD is multifaceted, encompassing genetic, environmental, and physiological variables. In spite of the existence of global health objectives, the incidence and mortality rates of COPD persistently escalate, exhibiting disparities influenced by factors such as gender, geographical location, and age. The increasing prevalence of COPD, therefore, necessitates a pressing requirement for enhancing treatment approaches and patient outcomes.

Keywords: chronic bronchitis, emphysema, respiratory, physiological variables, mortality

1. Introduction

Chronic obstructive pulmonary disease (COPD) is a prevalent and avoidable chronic respiratory condition. It is characterized by persistent obstruction of airflow in the airway, resulting from abnormalities in the lungs that are induced by harmful gases or particles [1]. The expiratory muscles responsible for generating contraction force, the elastic recoil pressure of the lung, and the airways are critical factors influencing the normal flow rate in healthy adults. However, individuals with COPD experience significant impairments in these factors, leading to a reduced quality of life [2]. The etiology of COPD is intricate, encompassing a diverse interplay of genetic, environmental, and physiological elements. The field of respiratory physiology, which encompasses the intricate mechanisms that regulate lung function, is of utmost importance in understanding the development and progression of COPD. The interplay at hand encompasses complex processes that involve structural changes in the airways, modifications in lung tissue elasticity, and dysregulation of immune responses. In 2012, the World Health Assembly introduced a health target known as the "25 by 25 goal." This objective sought to achieve a 25% reduction in premature deaths resulting from COPD and other non-communicable diseases by the year 2025. However, the global incidence of COPD has consistently risen, resulting in higher rates of morbidity, mortality, and overall disease burden. According to the GBD Chronic Respiratory Disease Collaborators [3], the global prevalence of COPD increased by 5.9% from 1990 to 2017. This period also saw the disease being attributed to a minimum of 2.9 million annual deaths. Based on projections made by the World Health Organization (WHO), it is anticipated that COPD will emerge as one of the top three leading causes of mortality on a global scale by the year 2030. The prevalence, mortality, and overall impact of COPD exhibit variations based on factors such as gender, geographical location, and age demographics. The incidence of COPD tends to rise with advancing age in the majority of regions. However, in certain regions, such as Uganda, the disease is more prevalent among children and young adults [4]. Despite the relatively low prevalence of COPD in certain Asian countries, such as India, the mortality rate associated with this condition remains alarmingly high [5]. COPD presents a significant disease burden in low-income countries, where healthcare resources primarily focus on addressing acute conditions like infectious diseases, rather than chronic ailments. Evaluating the COPD burden and identifying key risk factors across various levels can facilitate the identification of shared characteristics among high-risk areas and populations. This knowledge can provide valuable guidance for the efficient allocation of healthcare resources and the formulation of effective strategies for prevention and treatment.

2. Lung development and aging in the risk of COPD

The process of lung development is a meticulously coordinated event that commences during fetal development and continues throughout childhood and adolescence. Genetic and epigenetic factors play a crucial role in the intricate development of the respiratory system, which includes the branching airways and the complex alveolar network. Disruptions or insults experienced during crucial developmental periods can result in lasting structural changes that may increase the likelihood of respiratory diseases, such as COPD, in adulthood [6]. Differences in genetic factors related to the growth and maturation of the lungs, specifically involving the fibroblast growth factor (FGF) and transforming growth factor beta (TGF-β) signaling pathways have been linked to changes in lung development and heightened susceptibility to COPD in later stages of life [7].

The developmental origins of COPD have received significant attention due to the potential programming effects that arise from adverse fetal and early-life environments. Various factors, including maternal smoking, malnutrition, and exposure to pollutants, can influence lung growth and hinder typical structural development. Consequently, this influence can lead to compromised lung function and an elevated vulnerability to COPD during adulthood [8]. Furthermore, epidemiological studies have indicated a correlation between suboptimal lung function during early adulthood and an increased susceptibility to COPD later in life [9]. This highlights the significance of optimizing lung development as a strategy to mitigate the risk of COPD.

2.1 The interplay between aging and COPD

The process of aging is an unavoidable phenomenon that is marked by a gradual deterioration in physiological function across various organ systems, including the respiratory system. The susceptibility to COPD among older individuals is often attributed to age-related changes in lung structure and function, commonly known as "senile emphysema" [10]. The modifications encompass a reduction in lung elastic recoil, changes in chest wall compliance, and a decrease in the number of functioning alveoli. These factors collectively result in diminished lung efficiency and heightened susceptibility to airway obstruction [11].

In addition, the aging process is accompanied by a condition known as "inflammaging," which refers to chronic low-grade systemic inflammation. This systemic inflammation is characterized by elevated levels of pro-inflammatory cytokines, oxidative stress, and dysregulation of immune cells [12]. The phenomenon of inflammation is not limited to the respiratory system but rather affects the entire body. It has been identified as a contributing factor in the development of various age-related illnesses, such as COPD [13]. The presence of inflammation in older individuals contributes to an environment that promotes the continuation of inflammation and tissue damage associated with COPD, ultimately leading to an accelerated progression of the disease [14].

2.2 Genetic factors and risk of COPD

The influence of genetic predisposition on the risk of developing COPD has received significant acknowledgment. Evidence suggests that genetic variations in the genes responsible for encoding proteins involved in lung development, inflammation, and oxidative stress may contribute to an elevated vulnerability to COPD [15, 16]. Polymorphisms in the SERPINA1 gene, which encodes alpha-1 antitrypsin, and an increased risk of early-onset COPD [17]. The presence of genetic variations plays a role in the development of imbalances between proteases and antiproteases, ultimately leading to tissue damage and changes in immune responses [18]. However, genetic factors alone are not sufficient to cause COPD. Instead, they interact in complex ways with environmental exposures to influence the development and progression of the disease [19].

2.2.1 Environmental exposures

Environmental exposures play a crucial role in the development of COPD, as they result from the interaction between genetic factors and external triggers [20]. The inhalation of harmful particles and gases, particularly from cigarette smoke, continues to be a significant factor in the risk of developing COPD [21]. The inhalational insult leads to a series of events that involve inflammation, tissue remodeling, and oxidative stress, creating an environment that promotes damage to the airways and lung tissue [22]. Gene-environment interactions can increase the susceptibility to diseases, thereby enhancing the complex interplay between inherited vulnerabilities and external triggers [23].

2.2.2 Alterations in structure and function

The structural and functional changes within the respiratory system are essential in understanding the pathophysiology of COPD [24]. Chronic inflammation stimulate airway remodeling, which is characterized by increased production of mucus, thickening of the submucosal layer, and constriction of the airway lumen [25]. These modifications collectively contribute to the restriction of airflow and an increase in the effort required for breathing. Emphysema, a condition marked by the destruction of alveolar walls and loss of alveolar attachments, reduces lung elasticity and compliance. As a result, it negatively impacts both ventilation and gas exchange [10].

2.2.3 Immune dysregulation

An altered immune response is a key aspect of the intricate nature of COPD [26]. Resident immune cells, such as macrophages and neutrophils, contribute to the maintenance of chronic inflammation by releasing pro-inflammatory mediators [27]. The participation of T and B lymphocytes in the adaptive immune system contributes to the continuation of immune responses [28]. The complex immunological coordination is disrupted in individuals with COPD, frequently resulting in an imbalance between pro-inflammatory and anti-inflammatory pathways [22]. The exploration of modulating these immunological nuances presents a promising opportunity for therapeutic interventions [29].

3. The interplay between airway microbiome and the risk of COPD

The field of chronic respiratory diseases has experienced significant changes due to the study of the human microbiome, which refers to the extensive collection of microorganisms that inhabit our bodies. The study of the airway microbiome has become an intriguing area of research, providing valuable insights into the development and risk factors associated with COPD.

In the past, it was commonly believed that the lower respiratory tract lacked any microbial presence, while the upper airways were predominantly inhabited by bacteria that coexist harmlessly with the human body. Advancements in culture-independent techniques, such as high-throughput sequencing, have revealed a wide range of microorganisms present in the bronchial tree [30]. The airway microbiome comprises a diverse range of microorganisms, including bacteria, viruses, fungi, and other microbial entities. These microorganisms form intricate communities within the airway, displaying unique patterns that vary between states of health and disease [31]. The correlation between the prevalence of particular microbial taxa and the diversity of the airway microbiome has been observed with various respiratory conditions, such as COPD. A discernible disparity exists in the microbiome of the respiratory tract between individual with and without COPD. In addition, the composition of the microbiome changes exacerbations of COPD [32, 33], with notable variations observed among different subtypes of exacerbations [34, 35]. The aforementioned observations provide compelling evidence of a significant association between the lung microbiome and the underlying pathophysiology of COPD. This connection likely involves the interplay of host immunity and inflammatory responses. Dysbiosis, which refers to the disturbance of the microbiome, is thought to initiate an uncontrolled immune response in the host, resulting in heightened vulnerability to infections, inflammation, and negative impacts on the host's biology [36].

Typically, the airway microbiome in individuals who are in good health maintains a harmonious and well-balanced composition [37]. As airway diseases progresses, the microbial equilibrium is noticeably disrupted. Two primary metrics are utilized to measure microbial diversity, namely alpha-diversity (α-diversity) and beta-diversity (β-diversity) [35]. Alpha-diversity quantifies the overall diversity of microbial species present in a particular ecological niche, taking into account both richness (the number of taxonomic groups) and evenness (the distribution of abundances among these groups) [35]. In most lung diseases and instances of lung damage, α-diversity is notably decreased when compared to the airways of individuals with healthy lungs. In contrast, β-diversity quantifies the diversity of bacterial communities within a given ecological niche. As a result, β-diversity facilitates the evaluation of bacterial diversity across various ecological niches, such as the upper and lower airway, as well as different diseases. For instance, it allows for the comparison of the lower airway microbiome in patients with COPD to that of healthy individuals.

While the overall quantity of microorganisms in the upper and lower airways is comparable between individuals with and without COPD, there is a notable presence of dysbiosis in the lower airways of COPD patients [38]. A notable decrease in the diversity of the airway microbiome is primarily attributed to a reduction in the number of observed species. Additionally, the airway microbiome in COPD patients is characterized by a higher prevalence of bacteria from the Proteobacteria, Firmicutes, and Actinobacteria phyla, while the presence of bacteria from the Bacteroidetes phylum is comparatively lower [38]. At the genus level, the airways of individuals with COPD tend to harbor more bacteria belonging to the Hemophilus genus. Interestingly, although the Moroxella genus is seldom detected in the lower airways of individuals in good health, it is observed in the airways of approximately 2% of patients with COPD in their airways. The data collectively suggests that Hemophilus, Moraxella, and Pseudomonas are more abundant in individuals with COPD, whereas Prevotella is less abundant.

The α-diversity, specifically in species richness, decrease as the airflow limitation and burden of emphysema increases. However, this reduction is correlated with a concurrent decrease in the overall alveolar surface area [39].

4. Identifying risk factors for COPD

- Smoking: Smoking is widely recognized as the primary risk factor associated with the development of COPD. The majorities of individuals diagnosed with COPD are either current smokers or have a history of smoking. Individuals with a familial predisposition to COPD are at an increased likelihood of developing the condition if they engage in smoking behavior.

- Irritant: Additional lung irritants can encompass prolonged exposure to air pollution, chemical fumes, and environmental or occupational dust. Furthermore, inadequate ventilation when utilizing home cooking and heating fuels can contribute to lung irritation, as can exposure to secondhand smoke, which refers to the inhalation of smoke emitted by individuals who engage in smoking.

- Alterations to pulmonary growth and development: Pathologies impacting the respiratory system during prenatal development or early childhood can heighten the susceptibility [40].

- Infections: Certain infections, such as HIV and tuberculosis, are associated with an increased susceptibility to COPD.

- Age: The individual's age may contribute to their risk of developing COPD, particularly if they have other risk factors such as smoking. The onset of symptoms for individuals with COPD typically occurs in individuals aged 40 years or older [41].

- Alpha-1 antitrypsin (AAT) deficiency: This is a genetic disorder that elevates the susceptibility to COPD upon exposure to smoke, fumes, or dust. Alpha-1 antitrypsin (AAT) deficiency can also increase the susceptibility to COPD at an earlier stage in life [42].

- Asthma: Asthma is a respiratory condition characterized by inflammation and constriction of the airways. Approximately 20% of individuals diagnosed with COPD also present with asthma [43].

- Gender Differences: Gender is a significant factor in the risk of developing COPD, as research suggests that women are more vulnerable to the detrimental impacts of tobacco smoke and environmental pollutants [44]. The disparity can be attributed to hormonal factors, variations in lung anatomy, and differences in inflammatory responses.

- Socioeconomic Factors: The risk of developing COPD is closely associated with an individual's socioeconomic status. Individuals belonging to lower socioeconomic strata are at a higher risk of being exposed to environmental pollutants and occupational hazards. They also face limited access to healthcare resources and exhibit higher rates of smoking [45]. These various factors collectively contribute to an elevated risk of COPD among socioeconomically disadvantaged populations.

The aforementioned causes and risk factors have been found to elevate the likelihood of developing COPD. However, individuals residing in impoverished conditions and rural areas exhibit a higher susceptibility to COPD [46]. Additionally, COPD may exhibit varying impacts on women in comparison to men. In comparison to their male counterparts, older women may exhibit a higher propensity for experiencing severe symptoms of COPD, such as pronounced difficulty in breathing, despite having smoked less throughout their lifetime. Females diagnosed with COPD exhibit a higher propensity for experiencing symptoms at earlier stages of life and requiring hospitalization due to symptom severity, in comparison to their male counterparts with COPD [47].

Females diagnosed with COPD exhibit a reduced prevalence of smoking and possess a lower body mass index (BMI) compared to their male counterparts who are also afflicted with COPD [48].

The underlying factors contributing to the disparities in COPD prevalence and outcomes between males and females remain unclear. Researchers suggest that the cause could be attributed to hormonal or other physiological disparities between males and females [47–49]. Women have smaller lungs than men, which also may cause their airways to narrow those of more than men [50].

5. The significance of inflammation in the risk of COPD

Inflammation is a crucial physiological response to detrimental stimuli, intended to eliminate pathogens and facilitate tissue repair. However, in the context of COPD, the inflammatory process undergoes dysregulation and becomes persistent, thereby playing a significant role in the observed structural and functional abnormalities experienced by affected individuals. The key contributors to inflammation in COPD are immune cells, including neutrophils, macrophages, and T lymphocytes. These cells release various pro-inflammatory mediators, cytokines, and chemokines [51]. Additionally, it is worth noting that inflammatory mediators can also be produced by various lung cells, including epithelial cells. The primary inflammatory mediators comprise tumor necrosis factor-alpha, interleukin-1, interleukin-6, reactive oxygen species, and proteases.

The inflammatory process in COPD persists even after smoking cessation and continues to worsen over time. Hogg et al. [25] have demonstrated that patients with COPD experience progressive small airflow obstruction for several years following smoking cessation. The small airflow obstruction was caused by two factors: the accumulation of inflammatory mucous exudates in the lumen and an increase in the tissue volume of the bronchial wall. The augmentation of the tissue volume of the bronchial wall was distinguished by the infiltration of the wall by both innate immune cells (macrophages/neutrophils) and adaptive inflammatory immune cells (CD4, CD8, and B lymphocytes) that are organized into lymphoid follicles.

The precise determinants of inflammation in COPD following smoking cessation have yet to be definitively established. However, various factors, including autoimmunity, the presence of embedded particles/heavy metals from smoking, and chronic bacterial infection, have all been suggested as potential contributors [52]. Autoimmunity is widely recognized as the primary factor associated with lung inflammation in individuals with COPD.

The lung contains an intricate network of inflammatory mediators that are generated by both inflammatory and structural cells. These mediators encompass chemokines, growth factors, and lipid mediators. The factors that are most strongly linked to pathogenic inflammation in COPD include cytokines, reactive oxygen species, and proteases. The activation of toll-like receptors (TLRs) and lymphocyte antigen receptors triggers the production of inflammatory mediators. This process involves intracellular signaling pathways, such as nuclear factor kappa-light-chain-enhancer of activated B cells (NF-κβ) and signal transducers and activators of transcription (STATs), which ultimately result in the release of these mediators (**Figure 1**).

COPD is characterized by a significant systemic immune response, which becomes more prominent in the advanced stages of the disease and during exacerbations. Systemic inflammation is characterized by the presence of elevated levels of inflammatory/immune response mediators in the peripheral blood of individuals with COPD compared to smoking controls that do not have COPD.

The innate immune system serves as the initial defense against microbial infections, employing various cells (neutrophils, macrophages, dendritic cells, natural killer cells, monocytes, and mast cells) and humoral factors. These cells are equipped with pattern recognition receptors (PRRs), including Toll-like receptors (TLRs), nucleotide-binding domain leucine-rich repeat-containing receptors (NLRs), C-type lectin receptors (CLRs), RIG-I-like receptors (RLRs), and Interleukin-1 receptor (IL-1R) on their membranes. Cell apoptosis and necrosis triggered by stressors like smoking in individuals

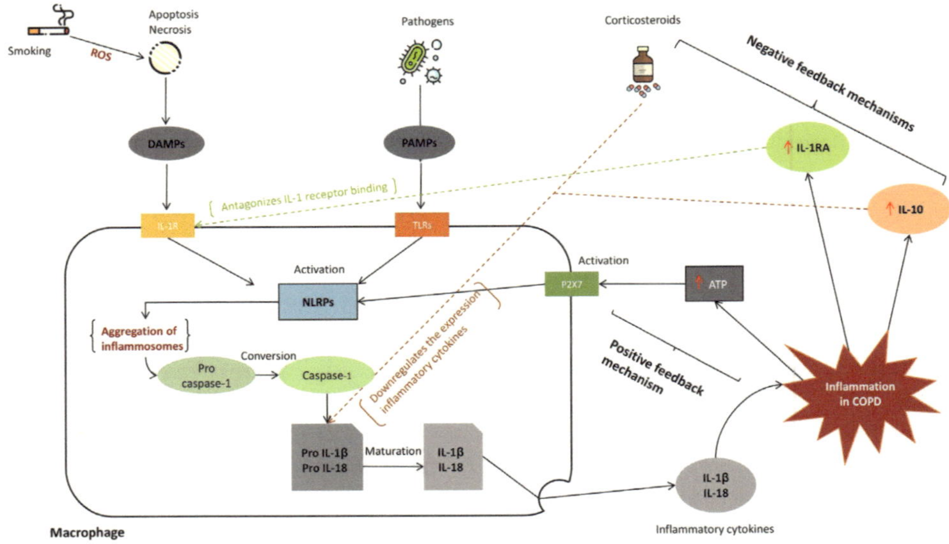

Figure 1.
The interplay of inflammatory process and COPD risk. The presence of embedded particles/heavy metals from smoking, and chronic bacterial infection activate cell recognition receptors (PRRs) like toll-like receptors (TLRs), nucleotide-binding domain leucine-rich repeat-containing receptors (NLRs), C-type lectin receptors (CLRs), RIG-I-like receptors (RLRs), and Interleukin-1 receptors (IL-1R). Stress-induced cell apoptosis and necrosis in COPD release damage-associated molecular patterns (DAMPs), recognized by IL-1 receptors, triggering inflammation. Microbial components release pathogen-associated molecular patterns (PAMPs) recognized by TLRs, activating NLRP inflammasomes. NLRP inflammasome activation leads to caspase 1 conversion, maturing pro-cytokines, exacerbating inflammation in COPD. The P2X7 receptor, elevated in COPD, activates NLRP inflammasomes, creating feedback loops of inflammation.

with COPD result in the liberation of molecules known as Damage-Associated Molecular Patterns (DAMPs). These DAMPs, recognized by the IL-1 receptor on immune cells, trigger inflammatory responses. In contrast, Pathogen-Associated Molecular Patterns (PAMPs) released by microbial components are recognized by TLRs, initiating a cascade of events in the cell. This cascade begins with the aggregation of NLRP inflammasomes in the cell due to activation of TLRs and IL-1R. Activation and aggregation of NLRP inflammasomes in response to DAMPs or PAMPs leads to the conversion of pro-caspase 1 to caspase 1, facilitating the maturation of pro-cytokines into their active forms. These active cytokines exacerbate inflammation in COPD when released from immune cells. Additionally, the P2X7 receptor, increasingly expressed in COPD, can activate NLRP inflammasomes upon binding with ATP, which accumulates due to heightened inflammation. This highlights a feedback loop where inflammation begets further inflammation in COPD as demonstrated in **Figure 1.**

6. The diagnosis and management of COPD

6.1 Clinical evaluation

The diagnostic process often commences with a clinical evaluation to identify symptoms. Frequent manifestations of COPD encompass persistent cough, production of sputum, dyspnea (characterized by a sensation of breathlessness), and wheezing.

The acquisition of a comprehensive medical history, encompassing aspects such as smoking habits and exposure to potential risk factors, is crucial in the process of diagnosing a patient.

The physical examination may reveal certain clinical manifestations such as diminished breath sounds, the presence of wheezing, and observable indications of respiratory distress.

Pulmonary function tests (PFTs) are a set of diagnostic procedures used to assess the functioning of the respiratory system.

Spirometry serves as the fundamental diagnostic tool and severity assessment measure for COPD. The test quantifies the forced expiratory volume in one second (FEV1) and the forced vital capacity (FVC). The ratio of FEV1 to forced vital capacity FVC is employed as a diagnostic measure to validate the presence of airflow restriction. One application of spirometry is post-bronchodilator testing, which evaluates lung function both before and after the administration of a bronchodilator. This procedure is valuable in distinguishing between reversible and irreversible airflow obstruction.

The combination of before and after measurements provides useful diagnostic information for the clinician that would not be known if only the measurement without bronchodilation were taken, specifically, the post-bronchodilator test which can help to:

6.1.1 Difference between asthma and COPD

The Global Initiative for Chronic Obstructive Lung Disease (GOLD) guidelines suggest that the diagnosis of COPD should be confirmed by spirometry. The presence of a post-bronchodilator FEV1 < 80% of the predicted value is indicative of COPD, while a post-bronchodilator FEV1 > 80% of the predicted value suggests asthma [53].

6.1.2 Assess bronchodilator responsiveness

A bronchodilator may be administered to assess responsiveness if an obstructive defect is present. The post-bronchodilator test can help to determine how much the bronchodilator medication helped with breathing. If the test shows that the airways have responded to the medicine, it can help to confirm a diagnosis of asthma [53, 54].

6.1.3 Treatment implications

- The diagnosis of reversible airflow obstruction indicates that bronchodilators and anti-inflammatory medications may be effective treatments. Clinicians can tailor the treatment plan to focus on managing airway inflammation and bronchoconstriction.

- The diagnosis of irreversible airflow obstruction suggests that the focus of treatment should be on managing symptoms and preventing disease progression. Smoking cessation and other interventions to slow down the structural changes in the airways may be prioritized.

6.2 Imaging

Chest radiography: Radiographic imaging of the chest may demonstrate signs of hyperinflation, flattened diaphragms, or other pathological findings.

Chest computed tomography (CT) scans offer a comprehensive evaluation of lung tissue, allowing for enhanced detection of conditions such as emphysema and bronchiectasis. These high-resolution scans give a more intricate analysis of the lungs.

6.3 The analysis of blood gases

The study of arterial blood gases (ABGs) aids in the evaluation of the levels of oxygenation and ventilation. Some of the gases measured in ABGs and the indicative range of values for each gas includes:

Partial Pressure of Oxygen (PaO_2).

Normal Range: 75–100 mm Hg.

COPD Implications: A decrease in PaO_2 is common in COPD due to impaired gas exchange in the lungs. As COPD severity worsens, PaO_2 levels may decrease. In severe cases, it can fall below 60 mm Hg, indicating severe hypoxemia (low oxygen levels).

Partial Pressure of Carbon Dioxide ($PaCO_2$).

Normal Range: 35–45 mm Hg.

COPD Implications: In COPD, elevated $PaCO_2$ (hypercapnia) is often observed, especially in more advanced stages of the disease. Increased $PaCO_2$ is a sign of inadequate ventilation and impaired CO_2 removal. A $PaCO_2$ greater than 45 mm Hg is indicative of respiratory acidosis, which is a sign of more severe COPD.

pH

Normal Range: 7.35–7.45.

COPD Implications: As $PaCO_2$ levels increase in COPD, the pH of the blood decreases, leading to respiratory acidosis. A pH below 7.35 is indicative of acidosis, which can be a sign of more severe COPD.

6.4 Alternative assessments

Testing for Alpha-1 Antitrypsin Deficiency should be contemplated in individuals presenting with early-onset COPD or those with a familial predisposition to the condition.

Electrocardiography (ECG) and echocardiography are diagnostic tests used to evaluate the presence of comorbidities such as corpulmonale, in which alterations in the pulmonary system lead to structural changes in the right heart.

7. COPD management

7.1 Smoking cessation

Smoking cessation: The act of quitting smoking is often recognized as the most impactful intervention in the therapy of COPD.

Behavioral counseling and pharmacology, such as the utilization of nicotine replacement therapy or prescription drugs, are frequently seen essential in the treatment process.

7.2 Pharmaceutical substances

Bronchodilators are a class of medications that are used to treat specific respiratory symptoms of COPD.

Short-acting bronchodilators, such as albuterol, are commonly utilized for immediate relief, in emergency situations, from some specific symptoms such as shortness of breath, wheezing, coughing and chest tightness.

Long-acting bronchodilators, such as long-acting beta-agonists (LABAs) and long-acting muscarinic antagonists (LAMAs), are commonly used as maintenance therapy. LABAs work by stimulating beta-2 adrenergic receptors in the smooth muscles of the airways. The activation of beta-2 adrenergic receptors causes relaxation of the smooth muscles surrounding the airways, leading to bronchodilation. This relaxation opens up the airways, making it easier for the individual to breathe. LABAs have a prolonged duration of action, providing bronchodilation that can last for approximately 12 hours, making them suitable for use as maintenance therapy.

LAMAs work by blocking the action of acetylcholine at muscarinic receptors in the airway smooth muscles. When acetylcholine binds to muscarinic receptors, it causes the airway smooth muscles to contract, leading to bronchoconstriction. LAMAs block these receptors, preventing acetylcholine from exerting its constricting effect, thereby promoting bronchodilation and improving airflow. LAMAs also have a prolonged duration of action, typically lasting 12 to 24 hours, which makes them also suitable for use as a maintenance therapy option.

Individuals who have frequent exacerbations or who exhibit an eosinophilic phenotype are advised to contemplate the utilization of inhaled corticosteroids (ICS). ICS are anti-inflammatory medications that can help reduce airway inflammation, including eosinophilic inflammation, and therefore, they can help control symptoms and reduce the frequency of asthma exacerbations.

The eosinophilic phenotype often refers to a specific pattern of airway inflammation characterized by an elevated number of eosinophils in the airway tissue and/or in sputum (mucus coughed up from the lungs). Eosinophils are a type of white blood cell, a part of the immune system. They play a role in the body's response to various infections and are also involved in allergic and inflammatory responses. Eosinophils are particularly associated with conditions involving inflammation of the airways, such as asthma. This type of inflammation is often seen in individuals who have allergic asthma, which is triggered by allergens, such as pollen or dust mites.

Eosinophilic airway inflammation can contribute to the symptoms and exacerbations of asthma, as eosinophils release substances that can cause bronchoconstriction (narrowing of the airways) and increase airway reactivity.

Eosinophil levels can be measured in different ways such as Blood test, sputum analysis and bronchoalveolar lavage (BAL).

Phosphodiesterase-4 (PDE-4) is an enzyme that plays a crucial role in the regulation of intracellular processes. Inhibitors may be employed as an adjunctive therapy in cases of severe COPD.

Antibiotics are indicated for exacerbations characterized by heightened sputum purulence.

7.3 Exercise

Pulmonary rehabilitation is a comprehensive program that aims to improve the overall well-being and functional capacity of individuals with chronic respiratory conditions.

Comprehensive interventions encompassing exercise training (such as pulmonary rehabilitation programs, physical therapy, and a home exercise plan), educational components (such as disease management education, breathing technique, and medication management), and nutritional assistance (such as dietary counseling and weight management) have been shown to enhance both the quality of life and exercise tolerance.

7.4 Oxygen therapy

Oxygen therapy is a medical intervention that involves the administration of supplemental oxygen to individuals with respiratory conditions or those experiencing low oxygen levels in order to improve their oxygen saturation and overall respiratory function.

The intervention was conducted on individuals exhibiting severe hypoxemia, characterized by a partial pressure of arterial oxygen (PaO_2) below 55 mm Hg or arterial oxygen saturation (SaO_2) below 88%.

7.5 Surgical interventions

Surgical interventions are medical procedures that use invasive techniques to treat or manage various health conditions. These interventions typically need the skills of trained surgeons, operating rooms equipped with specialized instruments, and the use of anesthesia to ensure the patient's comfort and safety during the procedure.

Lung Volume Reduction Surgery (LVRS) should be considered for a subset of patients who present with severe emphysema. The primary purpose of this procedure is to correct overinflated lungs and thus improve quality of life for individuals with advanced emphysema. While LVRS can be beneficial for many patients with severe emphysema, it is an invasive surgical procedure and carries certain risks, such as operative risk, pneumonia, air leaks, and pulmonary function decline and recovery challenges. It is therefore, necessary to take into consideration patient selection, pre-operative assessment, and post-operative management as crucial aspects of ensuring the success and safety of this procedure for those with severe emphysema.

Lung transplantation serves as a viable therapeutic option for those in the advanced stages of COPD. Due to some limitations such as donor organ availability, eligibility criteria, surgical risks, immunosuppression, rejection and complications, post-transplant care, cost and accessibility, and the complex nature of lung transplantation, it is considered as a treatment of last resort for individuals with advanced COPD.

Vaccinations are a crucial aspect of public health interventions aimed at preventing the spread of infectious disease.

The administration of influenza and pneumococcal vaccinations is effective in reducing the occurrence of exacerbations [55].

7.6 The management of exacerbations

While many of the above interventions are applied to treat COPD over the long term and to prevent the condition from worsening, patients with severe COPD have periodic exacerbations that require more acute treatment. In respiratory exacerbation, such as an acute exacerbation of COPD or asthma, several physiological changes occur in the airways, such as:

Airway Inflammation: Exacerbations are often triggered by increased inflammation in the airways. Inflammation leads to swelling and narrowing of the air passages, making it harder to breathe.

DOI: http://dx.doi.org/10.5772/intechopen.1003917

Increased Mucus Production: An overproduction of mucus in the airways can further obstruct airflow.

Bronchoconstriction: The smooth muscles surrounding the airways constrict, leading to narrowed air passages, which exacerbates the feeling of breathlessness.

Decreased Oxygen Exchange: These factors cause the exchange of oxygen and carbon dioxide in the lungs to become less efficient, leading to low oxygen levels (hypoxia) and high carbon dioxide levels (hypercapnia) in the blood.

The administration of bronchodilators, corticosteroids, and antibiotics is employed on an as-needed basis. The choice of treatment, whether it is bronchodilators, corticosteroids, antibiotics, or a combination of these therapies, depends on the underlying cause of the exacerbation.

Bronchodilators: Bronchodilators, like short-acting beta-agonists (SABAs) or LABAs, work to relax the smooth muscles around the airways, thereby alleviating bronchoconstriction and improving airflow. They are particularly effective when bronchoconstriction is a primary cause of the exacerbation, as seen in asthma or COPD.

Corticosteroids: Corticosteroids, such as oral or inhaled forms, are anti-inflammatory medications. They help reduce airway inflammation and swelling. They are useful when inflammation plays a significant role in the exacerbation, such as in asthma or some cases of COPD exacerbations.

Antibiotics: Antibiotics are used when a bacterial infection is suspected or confirmed. In some exacerbations, a respiratory infection, such as pneumonia, can be a triggering factor. If a bacterial infection is present, antibiotics are prescribed to treat the infection. However, they are not effective for viral infections.

Indications: Signs of a bacterial infection, such as increased sputum production, green or yellow mucus, fever, and changes in the appearance of chest X-rays, may lead to the use of antibiotics.

Non-invasive ventilation (NIV) is a therapeutic approach employed in instances of respiratory failure, and it differs from simple oxygen therapy and invasive ventilation (intubation) in several key ways:

7.5.1 Delivery method

NIV: NIV is delivered using a mask or other interface that covers the nose and/or mouth, or in some cases, a nasal mask. It assists with breathing by providing a combination of pressurized air or a mixture of oxygen and air. NIV is often administered using devices like bilevel positive airway pressure (BiPAP) or continuous positive airway pressure (CPAP) machines.

Simple Oxygen Therapy: Oxygen therapy involves delivering supplemental oxygen through various devices, such as nasal cannulas, face masks, or oxygen concentrators. It does not provide pressure support to assist with ventilation.

Invasive Therapy (Intubation): Invasive ventilation involves the placement of an endotracheal tube through the mouth or nose into the trachea, or a tracheostomy tube directly into the windpipe. It provides mechanical support for breathing by taking over the work of the patient's respiratory muscles.

7.5.2 Degree of intervention

NIV: NIV is considered a non-invasive and intermediate level of respiratory support. It does not require inserting a tube into the airway, making it less invasive compared to intubation.

Simple Oxygen Therapy: Oxygen therapy is the least invasive form of respiratory support. It simply provides additional oxygen to the patient without altering the patient's breathing pattern.

Invasive Therapy (Intubation): Intubation is highly invasive, as it involves the insertion of a tube directly into the patient's airway to take over their breathing completely.

7.6.3 Patient comfort and cooperation

NIV: NIV is typically well-tolerated by conscious and cooperative patients. They can talk, eat, and remove the mask when necessary. It is often used for patients with respiratory distress but who are still conscious and can protect their airway.

Simple Oxygen Therapy: Oxygen therapy is generally well-tolerated and does not interfere with a patient's ability to eat, talk, or move about.

Invasive Therapy (Intubation): Intubated patients are not able to talk, eat, or drink because the tube bypasses the vocal cords. Intubation requires sedation or even full anesthesia, and it is typically used for patients who are unable to protect their airway or breathe effectively on their own.

7.6.4 Indications

NIV: NIV is often used in conditions like acute exacerbations of COPD, congestive heart failure, or other forms of respiratory failure, where patients can still maintain some level of respiratory effort.

Simple Oxygen Therapy: Simple oxygen therapy is primarily used to correct hypoxemia (low blood oxygen levels) and is applicable in a wide range of respiratory conditions.

Invasive Therapy (Intubation): Intubation is reserved for patients with severe respiratory failure, inability to protect their airway, or who require complete control of their breathing, such as during surgery or when in a state of unconsciousness.

7.7 Interaction of different therapies

7.7.1 Combining therapies

Bronchodilators and Corticosteroids: It is common to use short-acting bronchodilators alongside inhaled corticosteroids (ICS) in the treatment of asthma and COPD. The bronchodilators provide immediate relief, while corticosteroids address underlying inflammation when used together in the form of a combination inhaler (e.g., LABA/ICS).

Bronchodilators and Non-Invasive Ventilation (NIV): During acute exacerbations of COPD or asthma, bronchodilators can be administered alongside NIV to help open airways and alleviate respiratory distress.

7.7.2 Patient-centered approaches

Individualized Treatment Plans: The choice of treatment often depends on the patient's specific symptoms, underlying condition, and severity of the exacerbation. For example, in COPD, some patients may benefit from inhaled bronchodilators alone for mild exacerbations, while others with significant inflammation may require corticosteroids in addition to bronchodilators.

Comorbidity Considerations: Patients with comorbid conditions may require tailored treatment approaches. For instance, a patient with COPD and heart failure may need therapies targeting both conditions simultaneously.

Response to Treatment: Patient response to treatments can vary. Some individuals may respond well to a particular therapy, while others may require a combination of interventions to manage their symptoms effectively.

7.7.3 Contraindications and cautions

Invasive Ventilation and Oral Corticosteroids: In some cases, when intubation and invasive ventilation are required, the use of oral corticosteroids might be reduced or stopped, as they can increase the risk of infections and complications.

Antibiotics and Viral Infections: Antibiotics are ineffective against viral infections. Using antibiotics when not indicated (e.g., in the common cold or uncomplicated upper respiratory infections) can lead to antibiotic resistance.

7.7.4 Escalation and de-escalation

Treatment Plans: The treatment plan may need to be adjusted based on how a patient's condition evolves. For instance, starting with non-invasive therapies like bronchodilators and corticosteroids and escalating to NIV or intubation if the condition deteriorates.

Prevention and Maintenance: Long-term management of chronic conditions often involves daily medications to prevent exacerbations. These can include inhaled corticosteroids, long-acting bronchodilators, and lifestyle modifications, alongside rescue medications for acute symptom relief.

8. Concluding remark

COPD represents a significant global health concern, warranting attention and concerted efforts on an international scale. Collaborative endeavors across nations have the potential to propel advancements in COPD research. The act of exchanging data, resources, and expertise has the potential to enhance the comprehension of COPD within various populations and facilitate the creation of interventions that are universally efficacious. Therefore, the advancement of research on COPD is crucial in order to boost patient outcomes and improve the overall quality of life for individuals affected by this incapacitating ailment. Future research should adopt the principles of precision medicine, harness the potential of artificial intelligence (AI) and big data, investigate innovative therapeutic approaches, and give precedence to the provision of patient-centered care. By acknowledging the diverse nature of COPD and customizing therapies to suit the specific requirements of each individual, researchers can make substantial advancements in combating this ailment, thereby enhancing the well-being of COPD patients on a global scale.

Author details

Patrick Godwin Okwute[1*], Adekunle M. Mofolorunso[1], Gideon Olamilekan Oluwatunase[2], Olayinka Olawale Asafa[3], Samuel Olalekan[4], Onome Bright Ogenetega[1] and Oyovwi Mega Obukohwo[5]

1 Department of Physiology, Babcock University, Ilisan-Remo, Ogun State, Nigeria

2 Department of Anatomy, University of Medical Sciences, Ondo, Nigeria

3 Department of Physiology, University of Ibadan, Nigeria

4 Department of Physiology, Olabisi Onabanjo University, Ago-Iwoye, Nigeria

5 Department of Physiology, Adeleke University, Ede, Osun State, Nigeria

*Address all correspondence to: patrickfavor.hp@gmail.com

References

[1] Soriano JB, Polverino F, Cosio BG. What is early COPD and why is it important? The European Respiratory Journal. 2018;**52**(6):1801448. DOI: 10.1183/13993003.01448-2018

[2] Okwute PG, Asafa OO, Eze U, Mofolorunso AO, Oluwatunase GO, Oghenetega OB. Postural alterations: Determinant of peak expiratory flow rate variation among young adults. Nigeria Journal of Biochemistry and Molecular Biology. 2022;**37**(2):133-137

[3] GBD Chronic Respiratory Disease Collaborators. Prevalence and attributable health burden of chronic respiratory diseases, 1990-2017: A systematic analysis for the global burden of disease study 2017. The Lancet Respiratory Medicine. 2020;**8**(6):585-596. DOI: 10.1016/S2213-2600(20)30105-3

[4] van Gemert F, Kirenga B, Chavannes N, Kamya M, Luzige S, Musinguzi P, et al. Prevalence of chronic obstructive pulmonary disease and associated risk factors in Uganda (FRESH AIR Uganda): A prospective cross-sectional observational study. The Lancet Global Health. 2015;**3**(1):e44-e51. DOI: 10.1016/S2214-109X(14)70337-7

[5] GBD 2013 Mortality and Causes of Death Collaborators. Global, regional, and national age-sex specific all-cause and cause-specific mortality for 240 causes of death, 1990-2013: A systematic analysis for the global burden of disease study 2013. Lancet. 2015;**385**(9963):117-171. DOI: 10.1016/S0140-6736(14)61682-2

[6] Hislop AA. Airway and blood vessel interaction during lung development. Journal of Anatomy. 2002;**201**(4):325-334

[7] Vestbo J, Agusti A. Pathophysiology, classification, and mechanisms of COPD. The Lancet. 2011;**378**(9804):1011-1023

[8] Hales CN, Barker DJ. The thrifty phenotype hypothesis. British Medical Bulletin. 2001;**60**(1):5-20

[9] Brändli O, Schindler C, Künzli N. Lung function in healthy never smoking adults: Reference values and lower limits of normal of a Swiss population. Thorax. 2003;**58**(8):733-740

[10] Hogg JC. Pathophysiology of airflow limitation in chronic obstructive pulmonary disease. The Lancet. 2004;**364**(9435):709-721

[11] King GG, Brown NJ, Diba C. The effects of body weight on airway calibre. European Respiratory Journal. 2010;**35**(5):1106-1113

[12] Franceschi C, Campisi J. Chronic inflammation (inflammaging) and its potential contribution to age-associated diseases. The Journals of Gerontology: Series A. 2014;**69**(Suppl_1):S4-S9

[13] Barnes PJ. Mechanisms and resistance in COPD: Nrf2 in the spotlight. Chest. 2011;**140**(3):560-565

[14] Vachier I, Bonnans C, Chavis C. Severe asthma is associated with a loss of LX4, an endogenous anti-inflammatory compound. Journal of Allergy and Clinical Immunology. 2005;**115**(1):55-60

[15] Silverman EK, Vestbo J. Agusti. COPD: The early years. The Lancet Respiratory Medicine. 2019;**7**(4):319-320

[16] Hogg JC, Timens W. The pathology of chronic obstructive pulmonary disease. Annual Review of Pathology. 2009;**4**:435-459

[17] Stoller JK, Aboussouan LS. A review of alpha1-antitrypsin deficiency. The American Journal of Respiratory and Critical Care Medicine. 2018;**168**(3):246-259

[18] Silverman EK, Sandhaus RA. Clinical practice. Alpha1-antitrypsin deficiency. New England Journal of Medicine. 2009;**360**(26):2749-2757

[19] Hersh CP, Hokanson JE, Lynch DA. Family history is a risk factor for COPD. Chest. 2010;**138**(1):39-49

[20] Eisner MD, Anthonisen N, Coultas D. An official American Thoracic Society public policy statement: Novel risk factors and the global burden of chronic obstructive pulmonary disease. American Journal of Respiratory and Critical Care Medicine. 2010;**182**(5):693-718

[21] Halbert RJ, Natoli JL, Gano A. Global burden of COPD: Systematic review and meta-analysis. European Respiratory Journal. 2006;**28**(3):523-532

[22] Barnes PJ. Mediators of chronic obstructive pulmonary disease. Pharmacological Reviews. 2004;**56**(4):515-548

[23] Siedlinski M, Cho MH, Bakke P. Genome-wide association study of smoking behaviours in patients with COPD. Thorax. 2013;**68**(8):769-777

[24] Cosio M, Ghezzo H, Hogg JC. The relations between structural changes in small airways and pulmonary-function tests. New England Journal of Medicine. 2004;**350**(26):2645-2653

[25] Hogg JC, Chu F, Utokaparch S. The nature of small-airway obstruction in chronic obstructive pulmonary disease. New England Journal of Medicine. 2004;**350**(26):2645-2653

[26] Agusti A, Hogg JC. Update on the pathogenesis of chronic obstructive pulmonary disease. The New England Journal of Medicine. 2010;**363**(23):2334-2345

[27] Barnes PJ. Immunology of asthma and chronic obstructive pulmonary disease. Nature Reviews Immunology. 2008;**8**(3):183-192

[28] Cosio M, Saetta M. Immunology of chronic obstructive pulmonary disease. Journal of Allergy and Clinical Immunology. 2006;**117**(3):551-560

[29] Rahman I, Adcock IM. Oxidative stress and redox regulation of lung inflammation in COPD. European Respiratory Journal. 2006;**28**(1):219-242

[30] Dickson RP, Huffnagle GB. The lung microbiome: New principles for respiratory bacteriology in health and disease. PLoS Pathogens. 2015;**11**(7):e1004923

[31] Marsland BJ, Gollwitzer ES. Host–microorganism interactions in lung diseases. Nature Reviews Immunology. 2014;**14**(12):827-835

[32] Sze MA, Dimitriu PA, Hayashi S. The lung tissue microbiome in chronic obstructive pulmonary disease. American Journal of Respiratory and Critical Care Medicine. 2015;**192**(4):438-445

[33] Sethi S, Evans N, Grant BJ. New strains of bacteria and exacerbations of chronic obstructive pulmonary disease. New England Journal of Medicine. 2002;**347**(7):465-471

[34] Segal LN, Blaser MJ. A brave new world: The lung microbiota in an era of change. Annals of the American Thoracic Society. 2014;**11**(Supplement_1):S21-S27

[35] Wang Z, Bafadhel M, Haldar K. Lung microbiome dynamics in COPD

exacerbations. European Respiratory Journal. 2016;**47**(4):1082-1092

[36] Shukla SD, Budden KF. Repeated sputum exposures do not alter pulmonary immune responses in COPD patients. Clinical & Translational Immunology. 2017;**6**(11):e159

[37] Hoggard M, Biswas K. Bacteriophage therapy for COPD. European Respiratory Journal. 2017;**49**(4):1700530

[38] Erb-Downward JR, Thompson DL, Han MK, et al. Analysis of the lung microbiome in the "healthy" smoker and in COPD. PLoS One. 2011;**6**(2):e16384

[39] Knudsen L, Ochs M. The micromechanics of lung alveoli: Structure and function of surfactant and tissue components. Histochemistry and Cell Biology. 2018;**150**(6):661-676. DOI: 10.1007/s00418-018-1747-9. Epub

[40] Grant T, Brigham EP, McCormack MC. Childhood origins of adult lung disease as opportunities for prevention. The Journal of Allergy and Clinical Immunology. In Practice. 2020;**8**(3):849-858. DOI: 10.1016/j.jaip.2020.01.015

[41] Dekhuijzen PNR, Hass N, Liu J, Dreher M. Daily impact of COPD in younger and older adults: Global online survey results from over 1,300 patients. COPD: Journal of Chronic Obstructive Pulmonary Disease. 2020;**17**(4):419-428. DOI: 10.1080/15412555.2020.1788526

[42] Senn O, Russi EW, Imboden M, Probst-Hensch NM. α1-antitrypsin deficiency and lung disease: Risk modification by occupational and environmental inhalants. European Respiratory Journal. 2005;**26**(5):909-917

[43] Knight A. Managing the overlap of asthma and chronic obstructive pulmonary disease. Australian Prescriber. 2020;**43**(1):7-11. DOI: 10.18773/austprescr.2020.002

[44] Aryal S, Diaz-Guzman E, Mannino DM. COPD and gender differences: An update. Translational Research. 2014;**162**(4):208-218

[45] Martinez CH, Mannino DM, Sood A. Socioeconomic indicators and COPD among non-smoking adults in the USA. Thorax. 2016;**71**(8):706-712

[46] Raju S, Keet CA, Paulin LM, Matsui EC, Peng RD, Hansel NN, et al. Rural residence and poverty are independent risk factors for chronic obstructive pulmonary disease in the United States. American Journal of Respiratory and Critical Care Medicine. 2019;**199**(8):961-969. DOI: 10.1164/rccm.201807-1374OC

[47] DeMeo DL, Ramagopalan S, Kavati A, Vegesna A, Han MK, Yadao A, et al. COPDGene investigators. Women manifest more severe COPD symptoms across the life course. International Journal of Chronic Obstructive Pulmonary Disease. 2018;**13**:3021-3029. DOI: 10.2147/COPD.S160270

[48] Zhang H, Wu F, Yi H, Xu D, Jiang N, Li Y, et al. Gender differences in chronic obstructive pulmonary disease symptom clusters. International Journal of Chronic Obstructive Pulmonary Disease. 2021;**16**:1101-1107. DOI: 10.2147/COPD.S302877

[49] Balthazart J. Minireview: Hormones and human sexual orientation. Endocrinology. 2011;**152**(8):2937-2947. DOI: 10.1210/en.2011-0277

[50] Chapman KR. Chronic obstructive pulmonary disease: Are women more susceptible than men? Clinics in Chest Medicine. 2004;**25**(2):331-341. DOI: 10.1016/j.ccm.2004.01.003

[51] Barnes PJ. Inflammatory mechanisms in patients with chronic obstructive pulmonary disease. Journal of Allergy and Clinical Immunology. 2008;**121**(2):413-423

[52] Han MK. Chronic obstructive pulmonary disease in women: A biologically focused review with a systematic search strategy. International Journal of Chronic Obstructive Pulmonary Disease. 2020;**15**:711-721. DOI: 10.2147/COPD.S237228. Erratum in: Int J Chron Obstruct Pulmon Dis. 2021 Nov 04;16:3017-3018

[53] Richter DC, Joubert JR, Nell H, Schuurmans MM, Irusen EM. Diagnostic value of post-bronchodilator pulmonary function testing to distinguish between stable, moderate to severe COPD and asthma. International Journal of Chronic Obstructive Pulmonary Disease. 2008;**3**(4):693-699. DOI: 10.2147/copd.s948

[54] Langan RC, Goodbred AJ. Office spirometry: Indications and interpretation. American Family Physician. 2020;**101**(6):362-368

[55] van Heuvel L, Paget J, Dückers M, Caini S. The impact of influenza and pneumococcal vaccination on antibiotic use: An updated systematic review and meta-analysis. Antimicrobial Resistance & Infection Control. 2023;**12**(1):70

Section 3

Diagnosis and Treatment

Chapter 3

Diagnosis and Management of Chronic Obstructive Pulmonary Disease

Abu Talha Hanfi and Sana Ahmad

Abstract

This chapter describes the chronic obstructive pulmonary diseases (COPD) its diagnosis, management and recent advances. Because it is third leading cause of death in world. It must be given more attention and discussion. COPD was broadly divided into Stable COPD, Infective COPD and Exacerbation COPD all of which have different management criteria. COPD is frequently misdiagnosed with other chronic respiratory diseases but the Global initiative for Chronic Obstructive Lung Disease score and the COPD assessment test score help to assess the disease. It is preventable and treatable diseases so the multidisciplinary approach should be followed so that the care of the patient is done in all the dimensions. Pulmonary rehabilitation is one of the advances and it shows major benefits for COPD patients.

Keywords: pathology, diagnosis, treatment, future directions, COPD

1. Introduction

In the recent definition given by Global initiative for Chronic Obstructive Lung Disease (GOLD), chronic obstructive pulmonary diseases (COPD) is defined as common, preventable and treatable diseases that is characterized by persistent respiratory symptoms and airflow limitations that arise from airway and/or alveolar abnormalities usually caused by significant exposure to noxious particle or gases. In high income countries the main risk factor of exposure is smoking and in low income countries, occupational exposure. COPD is a heterogeneous disease, but has a uniform GOLD definition in terms of lung function, exacerbation history and symptoms. The center hallmark of COPD is inflammation which plays a significant role in persistent changes in different sections of lungs. Another main risk factor for COPD is genetic predisposition and toxic exposure. COPD is thus a disease in which genetic abnormalities in combination of with the type and duration of exposures determine the clinical phenotype [1].

In COPD, chronic inflammations take place that lead to many structural and functional changes such as narrowing of the small airways and demolition of lung parenchyma, which results in loss of elastic recoil. These changes decrease the ability of the airway to open during expiration [2]. The main characteristic symptoms of the disease is airflow limitations and dysfunction in mucociliary function [3]. Several

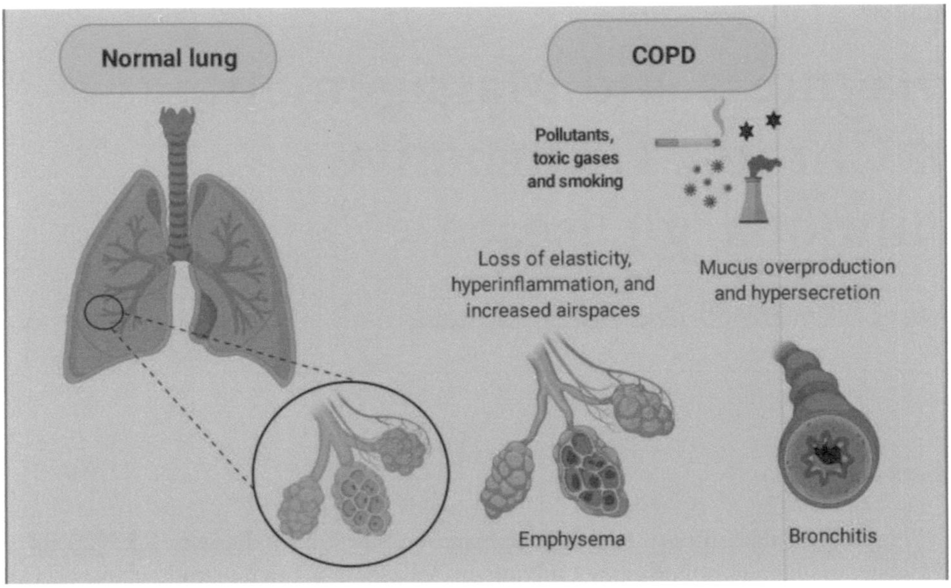

Figure 1.
COPD phenotypes which shows the structure of normal lungs and the abnormalities in COPD.

structural abnormalities present in COPD are shown in **Figure 1** Emphysema is defined as "destruction of gas exchange process on the surface of lung alveoli". Chronic bronchitis is an increase in the production of cough and sputum.

2. Prevalence

COPD is a highly prevalent disease, with over 250 million case worldwide presenting with severe chronic lung disease. Previously it was the fourth major cause of death globally, but in 2020 it was third. Recently it is observed that the prevalence of the disease is directly proportional to the consumption of tobacco smoking. The major risk factors for the prevalence of disease in many countries are occupational environment, pollution, and consumption of other biomass fuels. Therefore, it is predicted that the prevalence of the disease is increasing in the upcoming years due to aging of the population and exposure to these risk factors [4, 5].

3. Symptoms

The symptoms of COPD according to World Health Organization are shortness of breath, persistent cough, chest infection, wheezing, and weight loss and chest tightness.

4. Risk factors

4.1 Genetic factors

A genetic risk factor is a deficiency of alpha-1 antitrypsin (AATD). This deficiency is present in small portion of the world population, and it demonstrate the relationship between the genes and environmental factors that make an individual susceptible to COPD. Evidence suggests that a familial risk of airflow limitation is present in people who smoke and are sibling of patients with severe COPD [6].

4.2 Age and sex

Aging is associated with structural changes in parenchyma and in airways that may be associated with COPD. Most studies in the past have shown COPD is more prevalent in men, but recent studies show almost equal prevalence in men and women because of the consumption of tobacco smoking [7]. The prevalence of nonsmoking-related COPD is higher among women than among men. In the international BOLD study, among 4291 nonsmokers aged >40 years, 6.6% had COPD stage I and 5.6% had COPD stage II or higher [8].

4.3 Lung growth and development

The growth and development take place over extended periods, during the period of gestation, throughout childhood and into adolescence. Spirometer tests can reveal the increased risk of COPD and show that any factor that affects the growth of lung increases the risk of developing COPD. Lung infection during childhood is one of the contributing factors [9].

4.4 Socioeconomic factors

Lower socioeconomic status and poverty are associated with airflow obstruction, leading to increased risk of COPD. Reasons for the association include exposure of air pollutants, indoor and outdoor, infections and poor nutrition [9].

4.5 Exposure to particles

Cigarette smoking is the most common risk factor of COPD across the world. Compared to non-smokers, smokers have a greater chance of developing functional abnormality of lungs like decline in FEV1 values and other respiratory symptoms. Environmental tobacco smoke (ETS), commonly known as passive expose to cigarette smoke may also promote respiratory symptoms leading to COPD. When the smoking continues during pregnancy it also affects the growth and development of lungs of fetus. Occupational exposures to chemical agents, organic and inorganic, fumes, and other irritants are the risk factors of COPD. The high level of indoor pollution used for cooking in many houses such as that released from stoves that use wood, or animal dung typically increased the burden [10]. Among all smokers, 17.8% (1663/9169) had COPD (including incident and prevalent cases), whereas in never smokers the prevalence of COPD was 6.4% (318/4997). In men, 17.3% (n = 1042/6024) were never smokers, compared to 46.0% (n = 3955/8595) never smoking women. The proportion of COPD female cases without a smoking history was 27.2% (236/867), while the proportion of never smokers among COPD male cases was 7.3% (82/1126) [11].

4.6 Infections

Children who have a history of respiratory infections have reduced lung functional volumes and increased symptoms in their early adulthood. The infections play a susceptible role in exacerbation of COPD but development is not clear [12].

4.7 Chronic bronchitis

Chronic bronchitis was not directly associated with decline in lung functions. However, evidence shows association with hyper secretion and the FEV1 value of adults who smoke. The presence of diseases is associated with developing COPD [13].

5. Clinical manifestation

As shown in **Figure 2** the etiology of COPD includes smoking, pollutants, and other host factors, which leads to pathological abnormalities like emphysema and airway abnormality. These pathological abnormalities lead to increase in symptoms of COPD like airflow limitation, increase in secretion, and dyspnea [14].

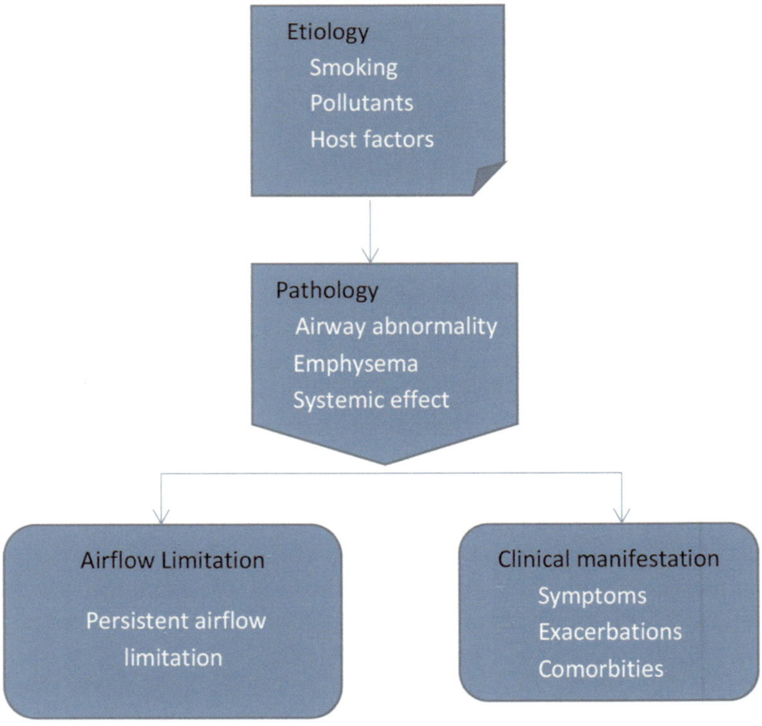

Figure 2.
The etiology and clinical manifestation of chronic obstructive pulmonary diseases.

6. Pathophysiology

Chronic obstructive pulmonary disease is characterized by many morphological and cellular changes that happen in the airways and in the lung parenchyma. These changes cause progressive airflow limitation by abnormal inflammatory reaction and poorly reversible airflow obstruction in the lungs. There may be inflammation in the lungs of cigarette smokers, but some of them have abnormal response of that agent that leads to COPD. As the response increases it leads to hypersecretion of mucous, called chronic bronchitis, and tissue destruction called emphysema and fibrosis.

As illustrated in **Figure 3** cigarette smoke and biomass fuel trigger the pathogenic changes such as inflammatory mediators, sub epithelial infiltration, CD-8 cells, CD-4

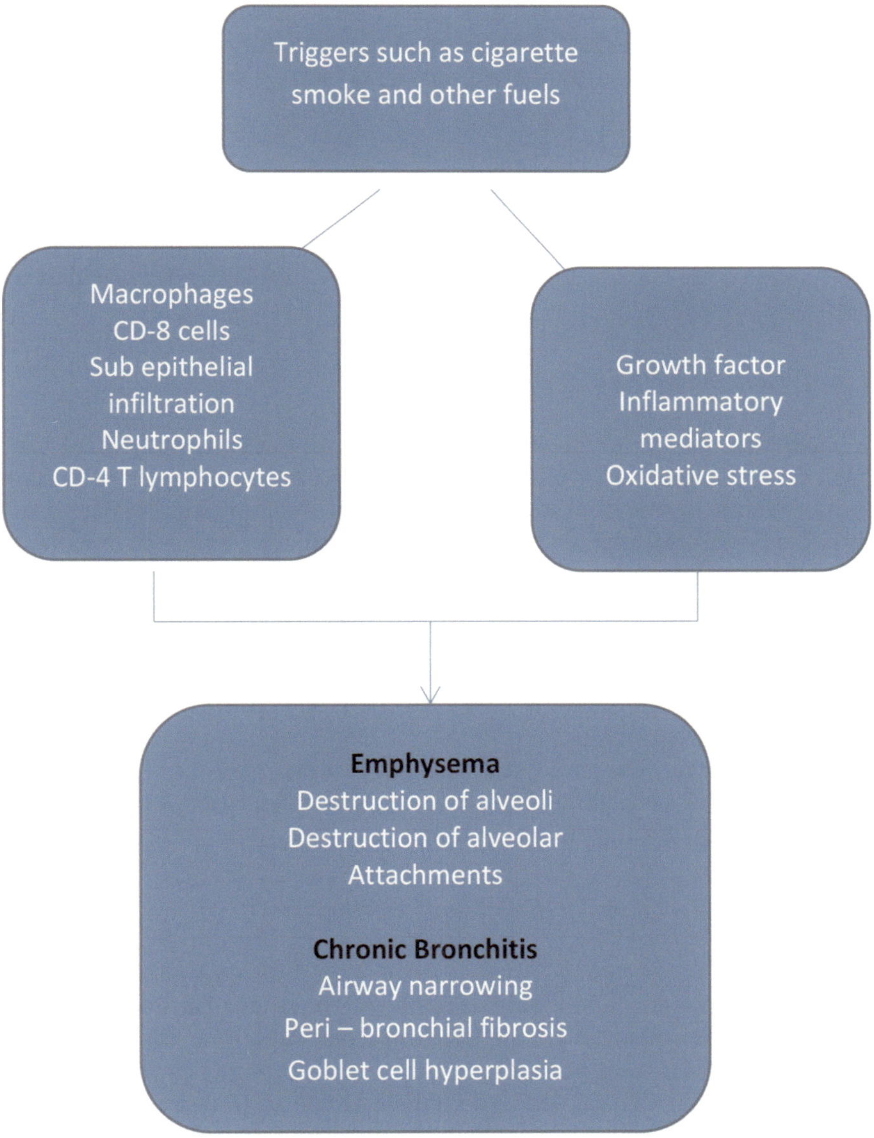

Figure 3.
Pathogenesis of COPD.

lymphocytes, macrophages and oxidative stress, which leads to destruction of alveoli, destruction of alveolar attachments, airway narrowing, goblet cell hyperplasia and peri-bronchial fibrosis. These pathologies are manifested by symptoms like dyspnoea, cough, and mucus hypersecretion.

Even after smoking cessations severity of the diseases can increase because many exacerbating structural and inflammatory changes have already taken place. Apart from inflammation, other processes take an active part in pathogenesis of COPD like imbalance between the proteases and antiproteases and oxidants and antioxidants (oxidative stress) in the lungs [15].

6.1 Inflammatory cells

Airflow obstruction in COPD is due to the increase in inflammatory cells such as neutrophils, T-lymphocytes and macrophages. Inflammatory cells release a variety of mediators and cytokines that promote progression of the disease.

6.2 Inflammatory mediators

Inflammatory mediators in COPD like macrophages and neutrophils produce Leukotriene B and T-cell chemoattractant. These agents amplify the pro-inflammatory response, and include CXC chemokines interleukin 8, and oncogene α, which is produced by epithelial cells.

6.2.1 Protease and antiprotease imbalance

An imbalance can occur between activation and production of proteases and reduction or inactivation of antiproteases. During cigarette smoke, the inflammation response produces an oxidative stress which releases a combination of proteases and in actives the antiproteases. Two main proteases are neutrophils, such as cathepsin G and proteases 3, and macrophages, such as cathepsins E, L, and S. Antiprotease includes secretory leucoprotease inhibitor, and tissue inhibitors of metalloproteases.

When an imbalance occurs between the proteases and antiproteases, alveolar wall destruction in emphysema and proteases causes mucous release. Increased oxidant from smoke releases chemostatic factors in turn directly affecting the mucous secretion and injury to alveolar walls.

As we discuss above, the pathogenic changes that are present in COPD causes many physiological abnormalities like air flow obstruction, mucous hypersecretion, pulmonary hypertension and ciliary dysfunction.

6.2.2 Airflow obstruction and hyperinflation or air trapping

The main factors of obstruction firstly occur in small airways of diameter less than 2 mm, because narrowing and inflammation flow into the small airways. Other factors contributing to airflow obstruction are loss of alveolar support and lung elastic recoil. The airway obstruction takes place due to increased trapping of air during the expiration phase of breathing that in turn hyper inflate at resting position and during exercise the trapping turns into dynamic hyperinflation. This process decreases the inspiratory capacity and lastly functional residual capacity results in breathlessness. The standard way of measuring the airflow obstruction to is by spirometry.

6.2.3 Mucous hypersecretion and ciliary dysfunction

Chronic productive cough is due to hypersecretion of mucous. The main characteristic of chronic bronchitis is mucous hypersecretion but not airflow obstruction. The irritation in the lung is by noxious particles, which result in hypersecretion due to increased size of sub mucosal glands, squamous metaplasia, and goblet cells.

6.2.4 Pulmonary hypertension

Pulmonary hypertension develops during progression of the diseases from abnormalities in the process of gas exchange. The factors leading to pulmonary hypertension are pulmonary arterial constriction and dysfunction of endothelium, and pulmonary capillary bed. In pulmonary arterioles, structural changes lead to right ventricular hypertrophy, pulmonary hypertension and cor pulmonale.

6.2.5 Gas exchange abnormality

Anatomical changes in COPD disturb the ventilation perfusion ratio—the main cause of gas exchange abnormalities. This disturbance is seen when progression of the diseases take place.

Despite significant progress over the last decade, COPD management has seen relatively few advancements. The existing medications do not considerably slow down the ongoing decline in airway function. Consequently, the main focus of treatment lies in enhancing lung function through bronchodilators and adopting healthier lifestyle practices. Since the airway obstruction in COPD is generally irreversible and current treatments do not change the course of the disease, the benefits of existing drug therapies are somewhat limited for patients.

7. Diagnosis and characterization

7.1 The GOLD score

The GOLD report categorizes COPD into four stages as follows,

7.1.1 Stage I: mild

FEV1 ≥ 80% predicted: the FEV1 value is greater than or equal to 80% of the predicted value for a person of the same age, sex, and height.

Symptoms: Mild airflow limitation with occasional symptoms such as chronic cough and sputum production. Shortness of breath may not be noticeable during normal activities.

7.1.2 Stage II: moderate

FEV1 50–79% predicted: The FEV1 value is between 50% and 79% of the predicted value.

Symptoms: Increased breathlessness during physical activities. Cough and sputum production are more noticeable, and exacerbation (worsening of symptoms) can occur.

7.1.3 Stage III: severe

FEV1 30–49% predicted: The FEV1 value is between 30% and 49% of the predicted value.

Symptoms: Further increase in breathlessness, reduced exercise tolerance, and more frequent exacerbations. Quality of life is significantly affected.

7.1.4 Stage IV: very severe

FEV1 < 30% predicted: The FEV1 value is less than 30% of the predicted value or FEV1 is <50% predicted with chronic respiratory failure (low oxygen levels).

Symptoms: Severe airflow limitation, extreme breathlessness even during minimal physical activity or at rest. Exacerbations, respiratory failure, and decreased quality of life are common.

7.2 The MMRC scale

In parallel with the GOLD score, the Modified Medical Research Council Dyspnea Scale is a tool used to assess the severity of breathlessness or dyspnea in patients with conditions such as COPD. It helps to understand the impact of breathlessness on a person's daily life and activities.

The scale provides a simple way for patients to describe their level of breathlessness.

The MMRC scale consists of five levels, each corresponding to a different degree of breathlessness:

1. Grade 0: Breathlessness only with strenuous exercise.

2. Grade 1: Breathless when walking up a slight hill or walking at a normal pace on level ground.

3. Grade 2: Walks slower than people of the same age on level ground because of breathlessness, or needs to stop for breath when walking at own pace on level ground.

4. Grade 3: Stops for breath after walking about 100 meters or after a few minutes on level ground.

5. Grade 4: Too breathless to leave the house or breathless when dressing or undressing.

This scale helps to understand the impact of COPD on a patient's daily activities and quality of life. It's used in conjunction with other assessments, such as lung function tests and symptom evaluations, to guide treatment decisions and monitor disease progression.

7.3 Spirometry

Spirometry is a crucial diagnostic test used to assess lung function and diagnose conditions like COPD. Spirometry findings in COPD typically show characteristic patterns associated with the disease:

1. FEV1:

    - In COPD, FEV1 is reduced due to airway obstruction and reduced lung elasticity.

    - A lower FEV1 value indicates more severe airflow limitation.

2. FVC:

    - FVC can also be reduced in COPD due to lung hyperinflation and air trapping.

3. FEV1/FVC ratio:

    - In healthy individuals, this ratio is typically high (around 80–90%) because they can exhale a large amount of air quickly.

    - In COPD, this ratio is reduced due to the airflow obstruction. It's a hallmark finding of the disease.

Based on the spirometry results, COPD can be classified into different stages according to the GOLD staging system:

- Stage I: Mild COPD—FEV1/FVC < 70% and FEV1 ≥ 80% predicted.

- Stage II: Moderate COPD—FEV1/FVC < 70% and 50% ≤ FEV1 < 80% predicted.

- Stage III: Severe COPD—FEV1/FVC < 70% and 30% ≤ FEV1 < 50% predicted.

- Stage IV: Very Severe COPD—FEV1/FVC < 70% and FEV1 < 30% predicted or FEV1 < 50% predicted with respiratory failure.

Spirometry findings, along with symptoms, exacerbation history, and other assessments, helps to guide treatment decisions and disease management strategies for individuals with COPD.

7.4 The CAT score

The COPD Assessment Test (CAT) is a questionnaire used to assess the impact of COPD on a patient's health status and daily life. The CAT questionnaire consists of eight items that cover different aspects of COPD-related symptoms and their impact. The total CAT score ranges from 0 to 40, with higher scores indicating a greater impact of COPD on the patient's quality of life. The scores are often categorized into four groups (A, B, C, and D) to guide treatment decisions and management strategies. These categories are determined by the total CAT score and the number of exacerbations experienced by the patient in the previous year.

Group A: low symptoms, low risk (CAT score < 10).

- Patients in this group have a relatively low impact of COPD symptoms on their quality of life.

- They are considered to have fewer symptoms and a lower risk of exacerbations.
- Treatment may focus on relieving symptoms, improving exercise tolerance, and promoting overall well-being.

Group B: high symptoms, low risk (CAT score ≥ 10).

- Patients in this group have a higher impact of COPD symptoms on their quality of life.
- They are still considered to have a lower risk of exacerbations.
- Treatment may involve bronchodilators and other medications to manage symptoms and improve lung function.

Group C: low symptoms, high risk (CAT score < 10).

- Patients in this group have fewer symptoms, but their risk of exacerbations is higher due to factors such as frequent exacerbations in the past.
- Treatment may focus on reducing the risk of exacerbations through interventions like long-acting bronchodilators, inhaled corticosteroids, or other appropriate medications.

Group D: high symptoms, high risk (CAT score ≥ 10).

- Patients in this group experience a significant impact of COPD symptoms on their quality of life and have a higher risk of exacerbations.
- Treatment may involve a combination of bronchodilators, inhaled corticosteroids, and other medications to manage symptoms and reduce the risk of exacerbations.

The CAT score categories help healthcare providers tailor treatment plans to individual patient needs, with the goal of improving symptoms, quality of life, and overall disease management.

7.5 Chest X-ray

Chest X-rays can exhibit the following indicators of COPD:

1. Hyper inflated lungs with flattened diaphragm.
2. Increased lung markings.
3. Narrowed heart shadow or flattening of the heart.
4. Bullae within the lung tissue.
5. Increased retrosternal airspace.

8. Risk factors and prevention strategies in COPD

In this section, we delve into the intricate web of risk factors associated with (COPD) and explore strategies to prevent its development. Understanding the interplay between genetic predisposition and environmental influences is crucial in deciphering the roots of this complex disease.

8.1 Environmental risk factors

We start by dissecting the crucial role of environmental factors. In developed nations, the chief contributor to COPD is cigarette smoking, whereas in developing countries, exposure to environmental pollutants like particulates from cooking with biomass fuels in confined spaces emerges as a significant trigger. Surprisingly, even among non-smokers, COPD accounts for a substantial portion of cases, suggesting diverse causes. Some instances stem from asthma evolving into COPD, identified by early onset and a history of variable symptoms. In countries like India, where biomass fuel exposure is prevalent, particularly among women, it becomes a major COPD risk factor.

Air pollution, certain workplace chemicals, such as cadmium, and passive smoking also amplify risk. The exact role of airway hyper-responsiveness and allergy in COPD remains uncertain. Nutrition, particularly during fetal life, plays a role—low birth weight leads to smaller lungs and earlier lung function decline. Early chest infections and latent virus infections like adenovirus might also influence COPD development. The connection between COPD and tuberculosis adds complexity to the picture [16].

8.2 Preventing environmental risks

A cornerstone of COPD prevention lies in avoiding environmental risks. Foremost attention is directed towards curbing smoking.

8.3 Smoking cessation

The act of quitting smoking yields the most rewarding outcomes. It not only slows down lung function decline but also curtails exacerbations and cardiovascular risks. Stopping smoking is most effective early in the disease and slightly less so as COPD advances.

Nicotine addiction complicates quitting, which should be seen as a remedy for drug addiction. Abrupt cessation often trumps gradual reduction, although, even after intensive programs, 75% of smokers remain at it a year later. Various methods aid in cessation: psychological counseling, group therapy, and nicotine replacement therapy (available as gum, patches, nasal spray, and inhalers). Bupropion, an unconventional antidepressant, and varenicline, a partial nicotinic agonist, show promise in aiding cessation [17].

8.4 Mitigating biomass fuel exposure

For those in developing countries, tackling COPD risk from biomass fuel exposure becomes pivotal. Alternative fuels like Liquefied Petroleum Gas (LPG) and natural gas, as well as improved stoves, improved ventilation, and cooking outdoors, offer preventive measures [18].

8.5 Genetic factors

Genetic predisposition's role comes to the forefront. Lung function monitoring in smokers reveals that a fraction of patients develops significant airflow obstruction due to accelerated lung function decline—genetics likely play a role. Patients with alpha 1-antitrypsin deficiency manifest genetic susceptibility to COPD. Yet, these cases are relatively rare. Genetic associations with other forms of COPD are still being explored, but few conclusive links have emerged [19].

8.6 Genetic research

Advances in genetic research reveal intriguing insights. Polymorphisms in genes related to nicotine addiction and nicotinic receptors surface as potential susceptibility markers. Techniques like gene chips, proteomics, and gene expression profiling are being harnessed to unravel the molecular nuances behind COPD development [20].

In this chapter, we navigate the multifaceted landscape of COPD risk factors, drawing attention to genetic influences, environmental triggers, and innovative prevention measures. Understanding this interplay enhances our ability to mitigate the onset and progression of this debilitating condition [21].

9. Treatment

9.1 Bronchodilators

9.1.1 Bronchodilator effect

Bronchodilators form the linchpin of COPD treatment, even though their effect on lung function is relatively modest in the context of COPD compared to asthma. Typically, they bring about around a 5% enhancement in FEV1, with some patients experiencing more substantial responses. Yet, their significance extends beyond this lung function improvement.

9.1.2 Beyond lung function

Bronchodilators have broader implications for COPD patients. They can alleviate shortness of breath and enhance exercise capacity, even when spirometry results show limited improvement. By reducing lung volumes, they mitigate hyperinflation, a condition marked by trapped air. This reduction in trapped air can lead to improved breathing during exercise and day-to-day activities. Additionally, bronchodilators might aid in reducing fatigue in respiratory muscles (although this is debated) and enhancing the clearing of mucus from the airways.

9.1.3 Choices in bronchodilators

Selecting the right bronchodilator hinges on patient preferences and cost considerations. Options encompass both short and long-acting beta-2 agonists, anticholinergics (muscarinic receptor antagonists), and high doses of theophylline. Notably, the spotlight rests on long-acting inhaled drugs, such as Long-Acting Beta 2-Agonists (LABA) like formoterol, salmeterol, indacaterol, and Long-Acting Muscarinic Antagonists (LAMA) like tiotropium bromide.

Long-acting inhalants are generally the preferred choice among bronchodilators. These drugs hold sway due to their sustained impact, offering benefits over an extended period. Formulations like LABA and LAMA have become favored choices in managing COPD, reflecting their efficacy in providing relief and improving lung function.

9.1.4 Wide spectrum of choices

The market offers a diverse range of bronchodilators tailored to the needs of COPD patients. Each holds unique features, and the selection process involves matching patient characteristics with the optimal bronchodilator.

This section uncovers the pivotal role of bronchodilators in of COPD management. From their impact on lung function to their potential to enhance overall well-being, bronchodilators stand as essential allies in the fight against the challenges posed by this intricate respiratory condition.

9.2 Anticholinergics: mastering airway control in COPD treatment

9.2.1 Origins and mechanism

The mechanisms through which anticholinergics are beneficial in COPD therapy are not yet fully elucidated. Initially, atropine, a natural compound, entered the scene for asthma treatment. Yet, due to its drying side effects, more soluble compounds like ipratropium bromide emerged. Anticholinergics, with their unique approach, rise as among the most efficacious bronchodilators for COPD. Notably, it is the vagal cholinergic tone that appears to be the only reversible element in the airflow obstruction seen in COPD [22].

9.2.2 Controlling airway tone

A subtle broncho-motor tone is present even at rest, thanks to tonic cholinergic nerve impulses. These nerve signals release acetylcholine near airway smooth muscles. Cholinergic reflex bronchoconstriction can be triggered by irritants, cold air, and stress. Anticholinergics come to the rescue by acting on small airways, minimizing air trapping, and consequently alleviating the burden of dyspnea and its symptoms.

9.2.3 Variety and efficacy

Notable anticholinergic medications like ipratropium bromide and tiotropium bromide are inhaled three to four times a day. On the horizon shines tiotropium bromide, administered once daily. The potency of tiotropium in enhancing lung function and quality of life spans all stages of COPD. Its efficacy remains impressive even when used alongside other therapies, as evidenced by the extensive UPLIFT study [23].

Remarkably, tiotropium brings a cascade of benefits, from reducing severe exacerbations and hospital admissions to curbing mortality due to COPD and cardiovascular disease [24].

9.2.4 Combination and tolerance

Anticholinergics and beta-2 agonists have synergistic benefits. Combining these treatments can offer additive bronchodilation effects. A blend of ipratropium and salbutamol in short-acting inhalers is popular. On the horizon, once-daily combination inhalers merging tiotropium with formoterol promise a new dimension in COPD care.

9.2.5 Safety and side effects

Safety considerations guide us in exploring anticholinergic tolerability. Inhalation of these drugs is well received, with systemic side effects remaining rare due to limited absorption. A unique highlight emerges as we dissect the effects of ipratropium bromide. Even in higher doses, it exerts minimal influence on airway secretions. However, nebulized ipratropium bromide, may trigger glaucoma in the elderly by affecting the eye directly. Notably, the implementation of a mouthpiece circumvents this risk. Dry mouth, a relatively common side effect, is observed in about 10% of that taking tiotropium bromide, seldom necessitating treatment discontinuation.

9.3 Beta-2 agonists

Beta-2 agonists serve as integral components of COPD management. Short-acting variants provide on-demand symptom relief, with the potential for regular use up to four times daily. However, LABA take precedence in COPD therapy, ensuring superior symptom control and maintenance. These agents exert multiple beneficial effects on the airways, inducing relaxation in both large and small airways by interacting with airway smooth muscle. Functioning as antagonists, they proficiently counteract bronchoconstriction, independent of its source. Experimental evidence reveals their prowess in reducing plasma exudation, reducing cholinergic reflexes, and even increasing mucociliary clearance when diminished. While not affecting chronic inflammation, they show promise in mitigating bacterial adherence to airway epithelial cells, potentially reducing infective exacerbations. Moreover, beta-2 agonists may amplify the ventilatory drive to hypercapnia, although the hypoxia response remains largely unchanged. Generally well-tolerated, side effects like muscle tremors, tachycardia, hypokalaemia, and restlessness occur with modest frequency. Importantly, excessive use does not appear detrimental, even in individuals with hypoxia and cardiovascular issues. Occasional hypoxemia may stem from a pulmonary vasodilatation-induced V/Q mismatch [25].

9.3.1 Short-acting beta 2-agonists

Short-acting inhaled beta 2-agonists (SABA) provide more immediate symptom relief. These agents include salbutamol and terbutaline. These agents are meticulously crafted to swiftly alleviate the burden of breathlessness and discomfort experienced by patients. Salbutamol and terbutaline take centre stage as potent solutions, designed to ease distress as required. An important consideration is that, regular usage may lead to the development of tolerance to their protective effects. Therefore, they are ideally used judiciously to avoid diminishing efficacy over time.

9.3.2 Long-acting inhaled beta 2-agonists

This section considers the use of the LABAs, salmeterol and formoterol in COPD management. With an efficacy spanning over 12 hours, these agents stand as defenders, providing sustained bronchodilation and guarding against bronchoconstriction. These agents are potent bronchodilators that also offer a range of benefits, from improved symptom relief, elevated quality of life, and enhanced exercise performance, to alleviation of airway obstruction in smaller passages. Illuminated by extensive long-term studies, their safety and ability to reduce exacerbations and even mortality underscore their vital role. The combined use of these agents with anticholinergics potentially leads to amplified advantages. Moreover, their interaction with bacterial adhesion sparks interest, raising the possibility of lowered infective exacerbations.

9.3.3 Oral beta-2 agonists

Oral beta-2 agonists provide an alternative avenue of relief for elderly individuals encountering challenges with inhaler use. While inhaled beta-2 agonists maintain preference, our focus shifts to the potential of slow-release oral preparations, including bambuterol and slow-release salbutamol. The advantages of these lie in their potential to target peripheral airways more effectively. However, this benefit comes with the trade-off of increased side effects compared to inhaled options. Central to this discussion is bambuterol, a prodrug that transforms into terbutaline, providing an effective once-daily regimen tailored for COPD management.

9.3.4 Theophylline

Operating in higher doses, theophylline's administration, particularly through oral means, showcases its potential to address the challenges of small airways, while also influencing mucociliary clearance and respiratory muscles. Recent insights reveal its anti-inflammatory capabilities, particularly in reducing neutrophilic inflammation in COPD patients. Theophylline's mechanisms encompass non-selective phosphodiesterase inhibition, elevated cyclic adenosine monophosphate (cAMP) and cyclic guanosine monophosphate (cGMP) concentrations, and adenosine receptor antagonism. Theophylline's potential in reversing corticosteroid resistance adds to its complexity. For practical implementation, theophylline finds a place as an additional bronchodilator, often considered for patients unresponsive to regular inhaled anticholinergics and LABAs. Recommendations suggest utilizing slow-release formulations twice daily to achieve desired plasma concentrations. As its anti-inflammatory and corticosteroid resistance-reversing properties come to light, theophylline's horizon in COPD management expands, potentially prompting the consideration of low-dose usage in conjunction with inhaled corticosteroids [26, 27].

9.3.5 Doxophylline

Doxophylline emerges as a methylxanthine akin to theophylline, boasting comparable bronchodilator attributes. Unlike theophylline, doxophylline stands apart as it refrains from adenosine receptor antagonism, mitigating concerns about cardiac arrhythmias or seizures. Moreover, the advantage of diminished drug interactions further enhances its profile.

9.4 Corticosteroids

The utilization of corticosteroids for COPD management remains a subject of ongoing debate. While the application of oral corticosteroids for maintenance treatment is discouraged due to limited benefits and substantial associated risks in the COPD population, inhaled corticosteroids are frequently prescribed at high doses under the presumption that COPD shares characteristics with refractory asthma. However, evidence supporting their efficacy in pure COPD cases is limited. Roughly 10% of COPD patients exhibit a positive response to oral corticosteroids, indicative of potential coexisting asthma; this subgroup may be better suited for regular inhaled corticosteroid treatment, recognizable through elevated eosinophil counts in sputum.

COPD patients generally show a subdued response to corticosteroids in contrast to asthma, with minimal improvements in lung function. While high-dose inhaled corticosteroids consistently exhibit a 20–25% reduction in exacerbations among severe cases, this stands as their primary clinical application.

The potential reduction in exacerbation frequency might be counterbalanced by systemic adverse effects like osteoporosis, especially among the elderly who may have inadequate nutrition and limited mobility. Indications of increased cataract occurrence and reported pneumonia among COPD patients are associated with high-dose inhaled corticosteroids, further adding complexity to their role. Consequently, the use of inhaled corticosteroids in non-reversible COPD remains uncertain, advocating for lower doses with reduced side effect risks; budesonide might offer a safer option compared to fluticasone propionate [28].

9.5 Combination inhalers

The integration of corticosteroids and LABAs in combination inhalers has garnered attention within COPD treatment, backed by various studies showcasing their advantages. However, the lion's share of benefits emanates from LABA component, with the combination's superiority over standalone LABA for reducing exacerbations potentially offset by escalated side effects due to corticosteroids [29]. Notably, combination inhalers not only ameliorate symptoms and curb exacerbations but also exhibit a discernible reduction in all-cause mortality, albeit narrowly missing statistical significance. The exacerbation reduction observed with twice-daily fluticasone/salmeterol approximates that of tiotropium, unveiling a comparable efficacy. These combination inhalers may prove invaluable for individuals with FEV1 less than 50% predicted, marked by frequent exacerbations (less than two per year), who are already on tiotropium and require supplemental treatment [30, 31].

9.6 Supplementary oxygen

Swift administration of controlled oxygen (24%) is pivotal in managing acute exacerbations, serving as a standard practice for hospitalized patients. Furthermore, Long-Term Oxygen Therapy (LTOT), also known as domiciliary oxygen, holds promise for specific COPD cases. Rigorous investigations through expansive multicentre trials have unveiled the life-extending potential of prolonged oxygen supplementation (less than 15 hours daily), manifesting a remarkable survival extension of approximately 30% in COPD patients. A cardinal objective of oxygen therapy is the elevation of PaO2 levels above the 60 mm Hg threshold or the attainment of an oxygen saturation exceeding 90%. However, caution prevails in pushing PaO_2 beyond the 60 mm Hg mark, as additional benefits become marginal while the risk of CO_2 retention escalates. Vigilant evaluation is indispensable before prescribing supplementary oxygen, as its use in patients with CO_2 retention warrants meticulous assessment to circumvent the peril of triggering respiratory failure [32].

9.6.1 Patient selection for Long-Term Oxygen Therapy (LTOT)

The criteria for LTOT suitability can be categorized as absolute and relative indications. The former encompasses scenarios such as

- Stable COPD over a three-week period under optimal therapy, coupled with hypoxemia and edema.

- FEV1 below 1.5 L and FVC below 2.0 L.

- PaO_2 below 55 mm Hg (<7.3 kPa)

- $PaCO_2$ exceeding 45 mm Hg (>6 kPa).

- Stability over a three-week period under optimal therapy is requisite.

- A relative indication is the need for palliative therapy.

The efficacy of portable oxygen should be gauged through the treadmill or six-minute walk test. Furthermore, individuals grappling with profound exercise limitations independent of oxygen desaturation may benefit from portable oxygen. This consideration extends to circumstances like commercial air travel, where the provision of portable oxygen is facilitated by the airline industry.

9.6.2 Provision of oxygen: diverse approaches and delivery methods

Diverse methods exist for furnishing supplementary oxygen, each tailored to specific circumstances:

Compressed gas cylinders: 100% oxygen stored in these cylinders necessitates frequent replenishment due to their bulkiness and weight. They are equipped with flow meters that offer either medium (2 l/min) or high (4 l/min) settings.

Oxygen concentrators: representing an economical and convenient choice for home-based LTOT, these devices stand as a practical means of oxygen delivery.

Liquid oxygen: carrying portability as an advantage, liquid oxygen is more expensive. Compact units weighing approximately 3 kg can provide oxygen for up to 14 hours at a flow rate of 2 l/min.

The avenues through which oxygen is dispensed include:

Face masks: while efficacious, close-fitting masks prove cumbersome and less suitable for prolonged usage due to discomfort.

Nasal cannula: commonly employed for oxygen delivery, these tubes are generally trouble-free. A flow rate of 1.5 l/min to 2.5 l/min is typically adequate to attain a PaO_2

exceeding 60 mm Hg (8 kPa). Supplement oxygen can cause nasal dryness and nasal irritation. Cold bubble humidification of low flow oxygen therapy via a nasal cannula did not produce any effect on the nasal mucosa and did not attenuate the oxidative stress caused by oxygen. However, it was able to improve nasal symptoms arising from the use of oxygen therapy [33].

Transtracheal catheter: Transtracheal Oxygen Therapy (TTOT) finds utility among select individuals unable to accommodate masks or nasal cannulas.

Pulsed delivery systems: incorporating technology like thermistors or pressure valves, these systems administer oxygen exclusively at the onset of inhalation. While costlier, they markedly curtail oxygen consumption by over one-third.

9.7 Antibiotics

Given that infection often triggers deterioration in COPD patients, effectively addressing infections through antibiotics is a crucial therapeutic aspect. Frequently, the organisms causing pulmonary infections are similar to those inhabiting the upper respiratory tract. Distinguishing if a pathogen in the sputum is the culprit behind exacerbation can be intricate, particularly as sputum color shifts to yellow or green during infection flare-ups, signifying empirical antibiotic initiation. Sputum purulence can result from neutrophil degranulation, which might not invariably signify bacterial infection. In fact, numerous COPD exacerbations likely stem from upper respiratory tract viruses, like Rhinovirus, Coronavirus, and Parainfluenza virus, making it challenging to differentiate between viral and bacterial origins [34]. The incidence of UTI increased over time in men and women with and without COPD. It was higher among men COPD patients than among non-COPD men [35].

While antibiotics are sometimes inappropriately employed, a meta-analysis of placebo-controlled trials for COPD revealed a minor yet significant Peak Expiratory Flow (PEF) discrepancy between antibiotic and placebo-treated patients. Notable bacterial culprits of COPD exacerbations encompass *Streptococcus pneumoniae*, *Haemophilus influenzae*, *Moraxella catarrhalis*, and occasionally *Mycoplasma pneumoniae*. Antibiotic selection hinges on likely pathogens, their community sensitivities, patient tolerance, and treatment response [36].

Preferred community treatments frequently involve amoxicillin or co-trimoxazole (Septrin), although the latter's use is discouraged due to resistance development and sulfonamide-related side effects. As many *H. influenzae* strains now produce beta-lactamase, curbing ampicillin/amoxicillin efficacy, initial therapy options often entail:

- Amoxicillin/clavulanic acid (Augmentin).
- Erythromycin or other macrolides (clarithromycin, azithromycin).
- A cephalosporin, e.g., cefaclor.
- A tetracycline, e.g., doxycycline.

Each drug presents pros and cons, and the optimal choice may depend on individual patient response, along with economic factors. Generally, amoxicillin, clavulanic acid, or doxycycline suffice for most ambulatory patients. Antibiotics should be administered at full therapeutic doses over approximately 10–14 days, with clarithromycin and azithromycin requiring shorter courses (3 days). Treatment cessation is warranted upon favorable response; inadequate responses might necessitate a switch to newer broad-spectrum agents like clarithromycin. Sustained antibiotic use is discouraged as it does not modify COPD progression and may foster antibiotic resistance [37].

9.8 Other drug therapies

Exploring mucolytic approaches in COPD management.

Mucus hypersecretion, a prevalent hallmark of chronic bronchitis, has prompted the exploration of various mucolytic therapies aimed at facilitating mucus expectoration, with the ultimate goal of potentially improving lung function. These approaches encompass a range of strategies, each with its own merits and limitations.

Stopping smoking, the most effective intervention stands as the cornerstone in mitigating mucus hypersecretion. Alongside this, anticholinergics have been investigated for their potential to reduce mucus hypersecretion, while beta-2 agonists and theophylline show promise in enhancing mucus clearance.

While certain drugs like bromhexol and ambroxol can decrease mucus viscosity in laboratory settings, their efficacy in improving lung function in COPD patients through controlled trials remains limited, leading to their exclusion as routine therapies. Similarly, expectorants such as guaifenesin and potassium iodide do not present proven beneficial effects.

9.8.1 Antioxidants

With the recognition of oxidant damage's potential role in COPD pathophysiology, antioxidant therapy has emerged as a logical avenue. N-acetylcysteine and carbocisteine initially designed as mucolytics, exhibit well-documented antioxidant properties. While initial meta-analyses hinted at NAC's efficacy in reducing COPD exacerbations by approximately 25%, large prospective trials have been less conclusive. A study in treatment-naïve patients from China revealed that carbocisteine demonstrated a reduction of approximately 25% in exacerbations over a year, suggesting a potential benefit for mucolytic/antioxidants in patients not on inhaled corticosteroids [38, 39].

9.8.2 Vaccines

Vaccination strategies offer a crucial defense against infections that trigger severe COPD exacerbations. Influenza vaccination holds significant importance due to its potential to reduce acute exacerbations and hospital admissions. Notably, evidence indicates reduced all-cause mortality in COPD patients following influenza vaccination, making it a cost-effective measure. Pneumococcal vaccination serves as a cost-effective method against pneumococcal lung infections, though large-scale trials for exacerbation reduction are inconclusive [40, 41].

9.8.3 Neuraminidase inhibitors

The application of neuraminidase inhibitors like inhaled zanamivir and oral oseltamivir in speeding up influenza recovery warrants attention. However, the specific impact of these inhibitors in COPD remains uncertain, as dedicated trials in this population are lacking, leaving the cost-effectiveness of this approach yet to be determined [42].

9.8.4 Antitussives

Cough, a frequently bothersome symptom in COPD, holds a potential protective role in facilitating secretion clearance. Consequently, the routine use of antitussives is not advised in the management of COPD (**Table 1**) [43].

Medications	Examples	Benefits	Side effects
Short Acting Beta-2 Agonist (SABA)	• Albuterol • Levalbuterol • Pirbuterol • Terbutaline	Bronchodilation rapid relief of symptoms, reduces anxiety, first-line rescue medications, alternative to oral steroids, portable and convenient	• Tremors • Nervousness • Headache • Tachycardia • Palpitations • Muscle cramps • Dizziness • Nausea • Insomnia • Irritation of the throat or mouth
Long Acting Beta-2 Agonist (LABA)	• Salmeterol • Formoterol • Indacaterol • Olodaterol • Vilanterol	Extended bronchodilation, reduced symptoms, improved lung function, enhanced exercise tolerance, decreased exacerbations, better quality of life	• Tremors • Tachycardia • Palpitations • Headache • Muscle cramps • Dizziness • Nausea
Oral beta 2 agonist	• Carbuterol • Pirbuterol • Procaterol • Bitolterol • Clenbuterol	Quick symptom relief, bronchodilation, improved airflow, exercise tolerance, reduction in anxiety, first-line rescue medication, combination therapy, easy to administer	• Tremors • Headache • Dizziness • Nausea • Changes blood pressure • Restlessness • Sweating • Palpitations • Digestive issues • Dry mouth
Long Acting Muscarinic Agents (LAMA)	• Tiotropium • Aclidinium • Umeclidinium • Glycopyrrolate • Revefenacin	Prolonged bronchodilation, improved airflow, reduced breathlessness, enhanced exercise tolerance, maintenance therapy, reduced exacerbations, convenient dosing, complementary to other COPD medications, better quality of life	• Dry mouth • Constipation • Urinary retention • Blurred vision • Dry eyes • Tachycardia • Headache • Sore throat • Allergic reactions • Bronchospasm (rare)

Medications	Examples	Benefits	Side effects
Theophylline	• Aminophylline • Theo-Dur	Bronchodilation, improved lung function, long-acting add-on therapy, reduced breathlessness, emergency use, potential anti-inflammatory effects, cost-effective, alternative for some patients	• Headache • Insomnia • Irritability • Nausea • Vomiting • Diarrhea • Restlessness • Tachycardia • Tremors • Dizziness • Palpitations • Changes in blood pressure • Increased urination seizure • High calcium levels • Difficulty urinating (elderly males with prostatism)
Doxyphylline	Brand Names • Doxolin • Duracron	Bronchodilation, symptom relief, reduced breathlessness, alternative to theophylline with potentially fewer side effects, option for patients who may not tolerate other bronchodilators	• Headache • Nausea • Vomiting • Insomnia • Epigastric pain • Irritability • Tachycardia • Tachypnea
Cortico-steroids	1. Inhaled cortico-steroids • Beclomethasone • Budesonide • Fluticasone • Ciclesonide 2. Oral cortico-steroids • Prednisone • Methyl-prednisolone • Prednisolone 3. Systemic cortico-steroids • Hydrocortisone • Methy-lprednisolone	Reduced airway inflammation, symptom control, exacerbation prevention, acute exacerbation treatment, enhanced response to bronchodilators, quality of life improvement, reduced hospitalizations	• Oral thrush • Hoarseness • sore throat • Skin changes • Cataracts • Glaucoma • Bone health issues • Adrenal suppression • Withdrawal symptoms
Combination inhalers	• Fluticasone/salmeterol • Budesonide/formoterol • Fluticasone/vilanterol • Fluticasone/vilanterol • Glycopyrrolate/formoterol • Aclidinium/formoterol	Improved bronchodilation, enhanced lung function, comprehensive symptom control, reduced exacerbations, convenient once-daily dosing, enhanced exercise tolerance	• Oral and throat irritation • Dry mouth • Tachycardia increased risk of pneumonia • Hoarseness and voice changes

Medications	Examples	Benefits	Side effects
	• Indacaterol/ glycopyrrolate • Tiotropium/olodaterol • Umeclidinium/ vilanterol		• Headache • Muscle cramps • Osteoporosis • Cataracts • Thrush
Oxygen therapy	• Target SpO2 85–88% and use appropriate oxygen delivery device according to it	Improved oxygenation, reduced shortness of breath, increased exercise tolerance, improved sleep quality, enhanced quality of life	• Dry or irritated nasal passages • Nasal congestion • Oxygen toxicity • Oxygen induced hypoventilation • Skin irritation • Claustrophobia
Antibiotics	• Azithromycin • Clarithromycin • Erythromycin • Amoxicillin • Doxycycline • Levofloxacin • Moxifloxacin • Ciprofloxacin	Infection control Reduction in exacerbation severity Faster recovery	• Nausea • Diarrhea • Abdominal pain • Allergic reactions • Rashes • Headache • Dizziness • Change in taste
Mucolytics	• N-acetylcysteine • Dornase alfa	Thinning and loosening of mucus Easier clearance of mucus from the airways	• Nausea • Vomiting • Stomach discomfort
Antioxidants	• N-acetylcysteine (NAC) • Alpha-lipoic acid (ALA)	Potential reduction in oxidative stress and inflammation	• Generally considered safe when taken within recommended doses
Vaccines	• Influenza (Flu) vaccine • Pneumococcal vaccine	Prevention of specific respiratory infections (e.g., influenza, pneumonia) Reduced risk of exacerbations in COPD patients	• Mild, temporary discomfort at the injection site • Rare allergic reactions
Neuraminidase inhibitors	• Oseltamivir • Zanamivir • Peramivir	Reduction in severity and duration of influenza symptoms, potential prevention of influenza infection in COPD patients	• Nausea • Vomiting • Headache • Dizziness
Antiussives	• Dextromethorphan • Codeine	Reduction in cough reflex Relief from dry, non-productive cough	• Drowsiness • Dizziness • Nausea

Table 1.
Summary of COPD drug treatment, benefit and side effect.

9.9 Non-pharmacological approaches in COPD management

9.9.1 Exercise

Physical exercise training, regardless of the specific type, is valuable for improving cardiorespiratory function in COPD. Both aerobic and upper limb exercises yield similar efficacy. Incorporating respiratory muscle training through resistive inspiratory loading can alleviate breathlessness, although comprehensive evidence from controlled studies remains inconclusive. Controlled breathing techniques like pursed-lip and diaphragmatic breathing show promise in reducing dyspnea, particularly in patients prone to hyperventilation [44].

9.9.2 Nutritional considerations

Nutrition is paramount in COPD management due to prevalent malnutrition and underweight status, though marked cachexia is now less frequent. Obesity may affect certain patients due to reduced physical activity. Addressing weight loss is crucial, especially for those with sleep disturbances, metabolic syndrome, or type II diabetes. Antioxidant vitamin supplements can also be beneficial. Nevertheless, high-fat nutritional supplements marketed for COPD have yet to demonstrate clear advantages [45].

9.9.3 Pulmonary rehabilitation

Rehabilitation endeavors to avert deconditioning and enhance the patient's capacity to manage their condition. Successful rehabilitation programs have proven to improve performance and quality of life, though not necessarily lung function. Patients with moderate-to-severe COPD are suitable candidates for pulmonary rehabilitation, encompassing educational guidance and physiotherapy. Notably, pulmonary rehabilitation synergizes with bronchodilator therapy [46].

9.9.4 Artificial ventilation

Remarkable progress has occurred in artificial ventilation devices. Nasal intermittent positive pressure ventilation has revolutionized COPD care, aiding both acute exacerbations management in hospitals and controlling hypercapnic respiratory failure at home. This technique ameliorates hypercapnia and respiratory acidosis, and grants rest to respiratory muscles. Positive outcomes have been noted, manifesting as reduced mortality and hospitalization periods during acute exacerbations [47].

9.9.5 Surgical options

For severe emphysema cases, various surgical interventions have exhibited success. Heart-lung transplantation, once predominant, has been largely replaced by single-lung transplantation in carefully chosen patients. Lung volume reduction surgery (LVRS) involving the excision of extensively affected emphysematous lung proves effective for selected individuals with primarily upper lobe emphysema and air trapping evidence. Patients without a barrel-shaped chest are significantly less likely to have airflow limitation.

LVRS yields sustained lung function enhancement, symptom reduction, and fewer exacerbations. However, very poor diffusing capacity increases mortality risk, underscoring the importance of patient selection. Recently, bronchoscopic lung volume reduction surgery methods have emerged to minimize the surgical complications of LVRS. Several devices, including valves, coils, and non-blocking techniques like bronchoscopic thermal vapor ablation and polymeric lung volume reduction, are currently under development to collapse and remodel hyperinflated lung regions [48].

9.10 Managing acute exacerbations

9.10.1 Preventive measures

A pivotal objective in COPD treatment is preventing exacerbations. Numerous interventions demonstrated through controlled trials to diminish exacerbation rates and hospitalization encompass long-acting bronchodilators (beta-2 agonists and anticholinergics), low-dose theophylline, high-dose inhaled corticosteroids, and smoking cessation.

9.10.2 Exacerbation implications

COPD exacerbations stand as a prime reason for hospital admissions. Beyond addressing underlying bacterial infection with antibiotics as previously discussed, exacerbations warrant symptomatic management, involving escalated doses of SABA and anticholinergic bronchodilators administered through nebulization. The role of antibiotics remains ambiguous due to limited clinical benefit in controlled trials, largely owing to the multifaceted origins of exacerbations, with over half stemming from viral or non-infectious causes.

9.10.3 Symptomatic management

To stabilize patients, oxygen administration (using a 24% or 28% Venturi mask) should attain a PaO_2 of at least 60 mm Hg without causing pH to drop below 7.26 (indicating acute alteration). Oxygen therapy's effectiveness should be assessed within an hour through blood gas analysis. Pulse oximetry may be employed for oxygen saturation monitoring, provided $PaCO_2$ and pH are within normal limits. Typically, a course of oral corticosteroids is recommended, marginally shortening in-patient stays by about 1 day. Extremely high doses of corticosteroids, like intravenous methylprednisolone, are usually unnecessary due to elevated side effect risks. Diuretics are suitable for peripheral edema. While chest physiotherapy may have value, evidence from controlled studies verifying its recovery-enhancing effect is scarce. Instances of rising $PaCO_2$ prompting respiratory failure might necessitate NIPPV or intubation.

9.11 Managing chronic disease

9.11.1 Accurate diagnosis and differentiation

Achieving an accurate diagnosis and distinguishing COPD from asthma is essential, typically discernible through patient history. Spirometry plays a pivotal role in objectively diagnosing airway obstruction and staging the disease, facilitating the selection of optimal therapeutic approaches. The GOLD guidelines delineate a stepwise escalation strategy for COPD treatment based on disease severity [49].

9.11.2 Foundational interventions

Throughout all stages, smoking cessation is paramount, especially in the early disease phases. Patients should routinely receive seasonal influenza immunization to mitigate complications. For GOLD stage 1, characterized by minimal functional impairment, treatment mainly involves as-needed inhalation of short-acting bronchodilators like salbutamol, ipratropium, or their combination.

In GOLD stage 2, a long-acting bronchodilator, such as tiotropium once daily or salmeterol/formoterol twice daily, is preferred. The once-daily regimen is often preferred by patients. If long-acting bronchodilators are financially unfeasible, regular administration of short-acting bronchodilators (e.g., salbutamol or ipratropium bromide), four times daily, or oral bronchodilators like slow-release theophylline or once-daily bambuterol, might be necessary. In some cases, a combination of long-acting anticholinergic and LABA is prescribed, preferably in a combination inhaler.

9.11.3 Advancing treatment

For GOLD stage 3 patients, the addition of inhaled corticosteroids (ICS) is considered, often through combination inhalers with a steroid and LABA. Additionally, oral theophylline may be introduced at this juncture due to its potential anti-inflammatory effects. Availability permitting, pulmonary rehabilitation could be beneficial. In GOLD stage 4, supplementary oxygen and, in carefully selected cases, lung surgery should be contemplated.

10. Conclusion

COPD is the most common respiratory diseases associated with high mortality and morbidity. There are many new treatment options present from oral pharmacological to surgical interventions that help the patient to improve the conditions. Pulmonary rehabilitation techniques are newer. A multidisciplinary approach helps the patient in an effective and efficient way. Continued advances in treatment should be made to improve the long term clinical outcomes and decrease the course of diseases.

Acknowledgements

I Abu Talha Hanfi wish to register my profound gratitude to Almighty for guidance and grace throughout my life. I would also like to extend regards to my amazing parents who are the source of success in my life. I would like to thank my wife.

The world is a better place to live. Thanks to people who want to develop and lead others. Thank you to everyone who strives to grow and help others grow.

Abbreviations

GOLD	Global initiative for Chronic Obstructive Lung Disease
COPD	chronic obstructive pulmonary diseases
AATD	alpha-1 antitrypsin deficiency
ETS	environmental tobacco smoke
FEV1	forced expiratory volume
MMRC	Modified Medical Research Council
FVC	forced vital capacity
CAT	COPD Assessment Scale
LABA	Long-Acting Beta 2-Agonists

LAMA	Long-Acting Muscarinic Antagonists
cAMP	cyclic adenosine monophosphate (cAMP)
cGMP	cyclic guanosine monophosphate
LTOT	Long-Term Oxygen Therapy
TTOT	Transtracheal Oxygen Therapy
PEF	Peak Expiratory Flow
ICS	inhaled corticosteroids

Author details

Abu Talha Hanfi[1,2,3,4]* and Sana Ahmad[5]

1 Symbiosis University Hospital and Research Center, Pune, India

2 Dr. D.Y Patil Medical College, Hospital and Research Center Pune, Maharashtra, India

3 Maharashtra Chapter—Indian Association of Respiratory Care (IARC), Maharashtra, India

4 Visiting Faculty at Symbiosis Institute of Health Sciences, Pune, Maharashtra, India

5 Royal Kalindi Hospital, New Delhi, India

*Address all correspondence to: abutalhahanfi@gmail.com

References

[1] Shrine N, Guyatt AL, Erzurumluoglu AM, Jackson VE, Hobbs BD, Melbourne CA, et al. New genetic signals for lung function highlight pathways and chronic obstructive pulmonary disease associations across multiple ancestries. Nature Genetics. 2019;**51**(3):481-493

[2] Gharib SA, Manicone AM, Parks WC. Matrix metalloproteinases in emphysema. Matrix Biology. 2018;**73**: 34-51

[3] Saetta M, Turato G, Maestrelli P, Mapp CE, Fabbri LM. Cellular and structural bases of chronic obstructive pulmonary disease. American Journal of Respiratory and Critical Care Medicine. 2001;**163**:1304-1309

[4] De Oliveira MV, Silva PL, Rocco PRM. Animal models of chronic obstructive pulmonary disease exacerbations: A review of the current status. Journal of Biomedical Science. 2016;**5**:2

[5] Mathers CD, Loncar D. Projections of global mortality and burden of disease from 2002 to 2030. PLoS Medicine. 2006;**3**(11):e442. DOI: 10.1371/journal.pmed.0030442

[6] McCloskey SC, Patel BD, Hinchliffe SJ, Reid ED, Wareham NJ, Lomas DA. Siblings of patients with severe chronic obstructive pulmonary disease have a significant risk of airflow obstruction. American Journal of Respiratory and Critical Care Medicine. 2001;**164**(8 Pt 1):1419-1424. DOI: 10.1164/ajrccm.164.8.2105002

[7] Hunninghake GM, Cho MH, Tesfaigzi Y, Soto-Quiros ME, Avila L, Lasky-Su J, et al. MMP12, lung function, and COPD in high-risk populations. The New England Journal of Medicine. 2009; **361**(27):2599-2608. DOI: 10.1056/NEJMoa0904006. Epub 2009 Dec 16

[8] Gut-Gobert C, Cavaillès A, Dixmier A, Guillot S, Jouneau S, Leroyer C, et al. Women and COPD: Do we need more evidence? European Respiratory Review. 2019;**28**(151): 180055. DOI: 10.1183/16000617.0055-2018

[9] Regan EA, Lynch DA, Curran-Everett D, Curtis JL, Austin JH, Grenier PA, et al. Clinical and radiologic disease in smokers with normal spirometry. JAMA Internal Medicine. 2015;**175**(9): 1539-1549. DOI: 10.1001/jamainternmed.2015.2735. Erratum in: JAMA Intern Med. 2015;175(9):1588

[10] Laumbach RJ, Kipen HM. Respiratory health effects of air pollution: Update on biomass smoke and traffic pollution. Journal of Allergy and Clinical Immunology. 2012;**129**(1):3-11

[11] Terzikhan N, Verhamme KM, Hofman A, Stricker BH, Brusselle GG, Lahousse L. Prevalence and incidence of COPD in smokers and non-smokers: The Rotterdam study. European Journal of Epidemiology. 2016;**31**(8):785-792. DOI: 10.1007/s10654-016-0132-z. Epub 2016 Mar 5

[12] Beran D, Zar HJ, Perrin C, Menezes AM, Burney P, Forum of International Respiratory Societies Working Group Collaboration. Burden of asthma and chronic obstructive pulmonary disease and access to essential medicines in low-income and middle-income countries. Lancet Respiratory Medicine. 2015;**3**(2): 159-170. DOI: 10.1016/S2213-2600(15)00004-1

[13] Gershon AS, Warner L, Cascagnette P, Victor JC, To T. Lifetime risk of developing chronic obstructive pulmonary disease: A longitudinal population study. Lancet. 2011; **378**(9795):991-996. DOI: 10.1016/S0140-6736(11)60990-2

[14] de Marco R, Accordini S, Marcon A, Cerveri I, Antó JM, Gislason T, et al. Risk factors for chronic obstructive pulmonary disease in a European cohort of young adults. American Journal of Respiratory and Critical Care Medicine. 2011;**183**(7):891-897. DOI: 10.1164/rccm.201007-1125OC. Epub 2010 Oct 8

[15] MacNee W. Pathology, pathogenesis, and pathophysiology. BMJ. 2006; **332**(7551):1202-1204

[16] Strachan DP, Seagroatt V, Cook DG. Chest illness in infancy and chronic respiratory disease in later life: An analysis by month of birth. International Journal of Epidemiology. 1994;**23**(5): 1060-1068

[17] Scanlon PD, Connett JE, Waller LA, et al. Smoking cessation and lung function in mild-to-moderate chronic obstructive pulmonary disease. The Lung Health Study. American Journal of Respiratory and Critical Care Medicine. 2000;**161**(2 Pt 1):381-390

[18] Fullerton DG, Bruce N, Gordon SB. Indoor air pollution from biomass fuel smoke is a major health concern in the developing world. Transactions of the Royal Society of Tropical Medicine and Hygiene. 2008;**102**(9):843-851

[19] Wan ES, Silverman EK. Genetics of COPD and emphysema. Chest. 2009; **136**(3):859-866

[20] Pillai SG, Ge D, Zhu G, et al. A genome-wide association study in chronic obstructive pulmonary disease (COPD): Identification of two major susceptibility loci. PLoS Genetics. 2009; **5**(3):e1000421

[21] O'Donnell DE, Fluge T, Gerken F, et al. Effects of tiotropium on lung hyperinflation, dyspnoea and exercise tolerance in COPD. The European Respiratory Journal. 2004;**23**(6):832-840

[22] Tashkin DP, Celli B, Senn S, et al. A 4-year trial of tiotropium in chronic obstructive pulmonary disease. The New England Journal of Medicine. 2008; **359**(15):1543-1554

[23] Decramer M, Celli B, Tashkin DP, Pauwels RA, Burkhart D, Cassino C, et al. Clinical trial design considerations in assessing long-term functional impacts of tiotropium in COPD: The UPLIFT trial. COPD. 2004;**1**(2):303-312. DOI: 10.1081/copd-200026934

[24] Wedzicha JA, Calverley PM, Seemungal TA, et al. The prevention of chronic obstructive pulmonary disease exacerbations by salmeterol/fluticasone propionate or tiotropium bromide. American Journal of Respiratory and Critical Care Medicine. 2008;**177**(1): 19-26

[25] Suzuki S, Watanuki Y, Yoshiike Y, et al. Effects of fenoterol on ventilatory response to hypercapnia and hypoxia in patients with chronic obstructive pulmonary disease. Thorax. 1997;**52**(2): 125-129

[26] ZuWallack RL, Mahler DA, Reilly D, et al. Salmeterol plus theophylline combination therapy in the treatment of COPD. Chest. 2001;**119**(6):1661-1670

[27] Culpitt S, Maziak W, Loukides S, et al. Effect of theophylline on induced sputum inflammatory indices in COPD patients. American Journal of

Respiratory and Critical Care Medicine. 1997;**157**:A797

[28] Brightling CE, McKenna S, Hargadon B, et al. Sputum eosinophilia and the short term response to inhaled mometasone in chronic obstructive pulmonary disease. Thorax. 2005;**60**(3): 193-198

[29] Calverley PM, Anderson JA, Celli B, et al. Salmeterol and fluticasone propionate and survival in chronic obstructive pulmonary disease. The New England Journal of Medicine. 2007; **356**(8):775-789

[30] Suissa S, Ernst P, Vandemheen KL, et al. Methodological issues in therapeutic trials of COPD. The European Respiratory Journal. 2008; **31**(5):927-933

[31] Davies L, Angus RM, Calverley PM. Oral corticosteroids in patients admitted to hospital with exacerbations of chronic obstructive pulmonary disease: A prospective randomised controlled trial. Lancet. 1999;**354**(9177):456-460

[32] Santana LA, Bezerra SKM, Saraiva-Romanholo BM, Yamaguti WP, de Fátima Lopes Calvo Tibério I, Dos Santos TM, et al. Cold bubble humidification of low-flow oxygen does not prevent acute changes in inflammation and oxidative stress at nasal mucosa. Scientific Reports. 2021;**11**(1):14352. DOI: 10.1038/s41598-021-93837-x

[33] Crockett AJ, Moss JR, Cranston JM, et al. Domicilary oxygen for chronic obstructive pulmonary disease. Cochrane Database of Systematic Reviews. 2000;(2):CD001744

[34] De Miguel-Diez J, Albaladejo-Vicente R, Palacios-Ceña D, Carabantes-Alarcon D, Zamorano-Leon JJ, Lopez-Herranz M, et al. The impact of COPD in trends of urinary tract infection hospitalizations in Spain, 2001-2018: A population-based study using administrative data. Journal of Clinical Medicine. 2020;**9**(12):3979. DOI: 10.3390/jcm9123979

[35] Walshaw MJ, Lim R, Evans CC, et al. Prescription of oxygen concentrators for long term oxygen treatment: Reassessment in one district. BMJ. 1988; **297**(6655):1030-1032

[36] Sethi S, Murphy TF. Infection in the pathogenesis and course of chronic obstructive pulmonary disease. The New England Journal of Medicine. 2008;**359** (22):2355-2365

[37] Saint S, Bent S, Vittinghoff E, et al. Antibiotics in chronic obstructive pulmonary disease exacerbations. A meta-analysis. JAMA. 1995;**273**(12):957-960

[38] Seemungal TA, Wilkinson TM, Hurst JR, et al. Long-term erythromycin therapy is associated with decreased chronic obstructive pulmonary disease exacerbations. American Journal of Respiratory and Critical Care Medicine. 2008;**178**(11):1139-1147

[39] Kirkham P, Rahman I. Oxidative stress in asthma and COPD: Antioxidants as a therapeutic strategy. Pharmacology & Therapeutics. 2006;**111**(2):476-494

[40] Bowler RP, Barnes PJ, Crapo JD. The role of oxidative stress in chronic obstructive pulmonary disease. COPD. 2004;**1**(2):255-277

[41] Schembri S, Morant S, Winter JH, et al. Influenza but not pneumococcal vaccination protects against all-cause mortality in patients with COPD. Thorax. 2009;**64**(7):567-572

[42] Schenkein JG, Nahm MH, Dransfield MT. Pneumococcal vaccination for

patients with COPD: Current practice and future directions. Chest. 2008;**133**(3):767-774

[43] Williamson JC, Pegram PS. Neuraminidase inhibitors in patients with underlying airways disease. American Journal of Respiratory Medicine. 2002;**1**(2):85-90

[44] Irwin RS, Boulet LP, Cloutier MM, et al. Managing cough as a defense mechanism and as a symptom. A consensus panel report of the American College of Chest Physicians. Chest. 1998; **114**(2 Suppl Managing):133S-181S

[45] Smith K, Cook D, Guyatt GH, et al. Respiratory muscle training in chronic airflow limitation: A meta- analysis. The American Review of Respiratory Disease. 1992;**145**(3):533-539

[46] Sharma S, Arneja A, McLean L, et al. Anabolic steroids in COPD: A review and preliminary results of a randomized trial. Chronic Respiratory Disease. 2008;**5**(3): 169-176

[47] Casaburi R, Kukafka D, Cooper CB, et al. Improvement in exercise tolerance with the combination of tiotropium and pulmonary rehabilitation in patients with COPD. Chest. 2005;**127**(3):809-817

[48] Kolodziej MA, Jensen L, Rowe B, et al. Systematic review of noninvasive positive pressure ventilation in severe stable COPD. The European Respiratory Journal. 2007;**30**(2):293-306

[49] Patel N, DeCamp M, Criner GJ. Lung transplantation and lung volume reduction surgery versus transplantation in chronic obstructive pulmonary disease. Proceedings of the American Thoracic Society. 2008;**5**(4):447-453

Chapter 4

Imaging of Emphysema: A Comprehensive Review

Karl Sayegh, Josephine Pressacco, Bojan Kovacina, Subba Digumarthy and Alexandre Semionov

Abstract

Emphysema is part of the chronic obstructive airway disease (COPD) spectrum, which also includes chronic bronchitis, asthma and bronchiectasis. Clinical differentiation of these conditions is often difficult, making imaging of paramount importance in correct diagnosis of COPD subtype. Imaging features of emphysema are reviewed in this article.

Keywords: emphysema, COPD, chest radiography, computed tomography, imaging

1. Introduction

Chronic obstructive pulmonary disease (COPD) is the 4th leading cause of death in the world, and one of the leading causes of morbidity resulting in substantial economic burden on healthcare worldwide [1].

COPD is characterized by persistent airflow limitation caused by a combination of small airway disease (obstructive bronchiolitis) and pulmonary parenchymal damage (emphysema). Although COPD can develop in non-smokers, cigarette and other types of smoking is the most common recognized risk factor in the development of COPD. Exposure to various organic and inorganic dusts, chemical agents and fumes, such as from coal and wood burning, together with genetic predisposition, lung development abnormalities, accelerated aging, bronchial hyper-reactivity and low socio-economical status are additional risk factors for development of COPD [1]. Cumulative exposure to inhaled noxious substances and other risk factors over decades is believed to induce a modified chronic inflammatory response and altered repair mechanisms in the lung, resulting in a cycle of repeated injury and repair in the airways, lung parenchyma and vasculature. Over time this may lead to progressive airflow limitation, air trapping and parenchymal destruction, despite cessation of causal agents, such as smoking [1].

Essential components of a clinical diagnosis of COPD are spirometry, presence of symptoms and exposure to risk factors. COPD usually presents as chronic and progressive dyspnea, cough and mucous production. Spirometry testing is required to confirm COPD diagnosis. A post bronchodilator ratio of the forced expiratory volume in 1 s (FEV1) to forced vital capacity (FVC) below 70% (FEV1/FVC < 0.70) is diagnostic of persistent airflow limitation. Post bronchodilator FEV1 is an indicator of the severity of airflow limitation and is associated with an increased risk of acute exacerbations and death [1].

Diagnosis of COPD based on clinical information, including spirometry data, does not distinguish among different subtypes of COPD, which comprise emphysema, chronic bronchitis, asthma and bronchiectasis. Emphysema is defined as "an abnormal, permanent enlargement of the airspaces distal to the terminal bronchioles, accompanied by destruction of the alveolar walls, without obvious fibrosis" [2], whereas the remaining COPD subtypes result in small airway disease. From an imaging perspective, these subtypes can however often be distinguished, although it is important to emphasize that different COPD entities may coexist. Furthermore, imaging often allows characterization of emphysema types, yielding a more precise diagnosis.

This review focuses on the appearance of various subtypes of emphysema on chest radiographs (CXR) and computed tomography (CT). Radiographic features of the pulmonary diseases are generally described in terms of the degree of attenuation of the x-rays, with high attenuation being white and low attenuation being black in conventional radiology images. "Opacity" and "shadowing" refer to areas that are less dark than normal lung parenchyma should appear. "Lucency" appears as darker areas.

2. Emphysema classification

Morphologically emphysema is classified into three major subtypes which can coexist: centrilobular, paraseptal and panacinar. Such classification takes into account the affected portion of the acinus – the terminal respiratory unit of the lung located distal to the terminal bronchiole. Additionally, emphysema in which the enlarged airspaces are over 1 cm in diameter is referred to as "bullous emphysema". Each of these subtypes is associated with underlying causes, as shown in **Table 1**. Distinguishing these subtypes is easier by CT than chest radiography, but becomes more challenging in advanced stages of the disease, even by CT.

Centrilobular or centriacinar emphysema is the most common type of emphysema and the one most associated with cigarette smoking. Pathologically, the central portion of the acinus (i.e. the proximal respiratory bronchioles and their associated alveoli) is destroyed [3]. On CT, centrilobular emphysema may appear to arise from the center of the secondary pulmonary lobule [4]. It usually affects the upper lobes and superior segments of the lower lobes, with the central lung being more affected than the periphery. The reasons for this distribution are not fully understood and may include differential perfusion, immunological make-up, dust clearance mechanisms, pleural pressure and lymphatic flow of the affected regions.

Mild-to-moderate centrilobular emphysema is characterized by multiple round or oval low-attenuation areas, usually several millimeters in size, predominantly scattered in the upper and inner lung zones (**Figure 1**). These small areas of low attenuation have no definable walls (as opposed to lung cysts) and are bordered by normal lung parenchyma; however they may coalesce and form larger lucencies, with well-defined and thin walls formed by compressed adjacent lung parenchyma separating them from normal lung parenchyma [5].

Although severe centrilobular emphysema may be difficult to distinguish from other subtypes, its distribution is helpful in differentiating it from panacinar emphysema (**Figure 2**). Also the presence of preserved lung parenchyma around large airways and vessels, anatomically located in the perilobular portion of the

Underlying cause Type of Emphysema	Tobacco Smoking	Connective tissue disorders	Alpha 1-Antitrypsin deficiency	IV talc injection	Heroin, cocaine and cannabis smoking	Hypo-complementemic Urticarial Vasculitis syndrome
Centrilobular	√					
Paraseptal	√	√			√	
Panacinar			√	√		√

Table 1.
Different types of emphysema versus underlying cause.

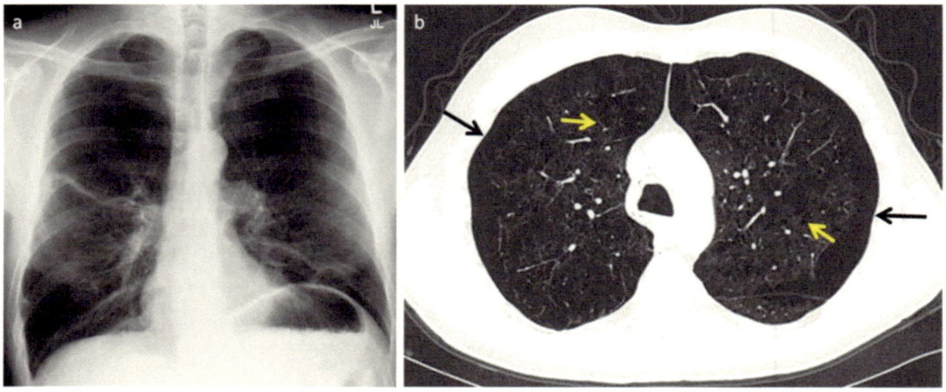

Figure 1.
Forty nine year-old male with prior history of smoking (35 pack-year) and exposure to distillates and nickel in pharmaceutical lab with centrilobular and paraseptal emphysema. (a) PA CXR shows increased lucency bilaterally predominantly in the upper lung zones. Note the absence of vessels in the outer third of the lung in the bilateral upper lobes. Incidental note of a linear scar in the right mid lung. (b) Axial CT image allows better appreciation of the combined centrilobular and paraseptal emphysema. The areas of centrilobular emphysema appear as punched out lesions in the central portion of the lungs (yellow arrows). Notice the typical subpleural and upper lobe predominance of paraseptal emphysema (black arrows). Paraseptal emphysema is so severe that the subpleural interlobular septa are either not visible on this 1 mm thickness CT or partially destroyed. The patient subsequently underwent bilateral lung transplantation.

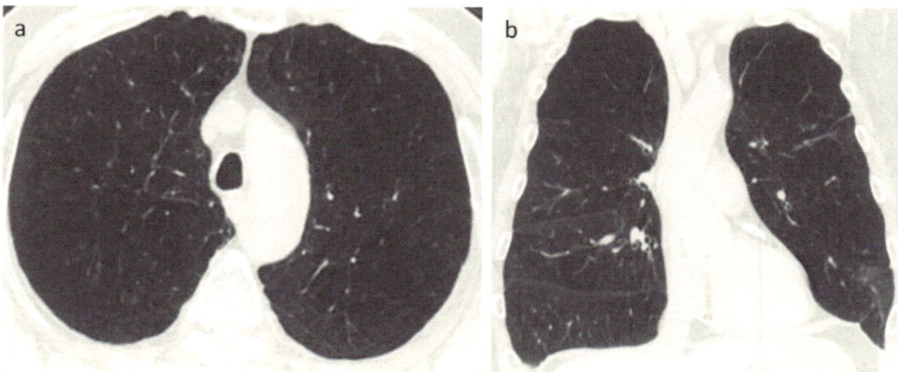

Figure 2.
Seventy nine year-old male with very severe COPD (FEV1 0.85 l, 29% predicted; FVC 2.9 l, 74% predicted; FEV1/FVC 29%. Axial (a) and coronal (b) CT images demonstrate severe centrilobular emphysema mimicking panlobular emphysema. The upper lung predominance is the best clue allowing to differentiate it from panlobular emphysema. Also note a lesser degree of hyperinflation compared to panlobular emphysema such as in cases of alpha-1 antitrypsin deficiency (refer to **Figure 5***). The destruction of the secondary pulmonary lobules is so severe that the attenuation of the lung in the left upper lobe is equal to that of the column of air in the trachea (−980 HU); this was confirmed by impaired gas exchange (DLCO 4.6 ml/min/mmHg, 20% predicted).*

secondary pulmonary lobule, is a clue that emphysema has originated in the centrilobular portion [4].

Distal acinar or paraseptal emphysema typically affects the subpleural upper lungs including perifissural and peribronchovascular lung parenchyma. This type of emphysema may not be associated with smoking and is usually not associated with airflow obstruction. Pathologically, the distal portion of the acinus – alveolar ducts and sacs, is destroyed. On CT, it is characterized by multiple subpleural and peribronchovascular areas of low attenuation, ranging from a few millimeters to 1 cm in diameter (with occasional bullae formation), separated by thin intact interlobular septa (**Figure 3**). It should be distinguished from honeycombing, which presents with much thicker walls, is multilayered, more frequent at the lung bases and is associated with fibrosis and architectural distortion [3]. Blebs and bullae can result in pneumothorax in young patients [3, 4] (**Figure 4**).

Panacinar or panlobular emphysema typically affects the lower lung zones and is usually seen in alpha-1 antitrypsin deficiency. Other causes of panlobular emphysema include Swyer-James syndrome and intravenous injection of talc-containing substances (usually in the context of illicit drug abuse). Pathologically, the entire acini, from respiratory bronchioles to alveoli, are uniformly enlarged [3, 4]. On CT, this appears as extensive areas of uniform low attenuation without sparing of any component of the secondary pulmonary lobule or acinus. This commonly results in a greater degree of lung inflation than in centrilobular emphysema [3] (**Figure 5**).

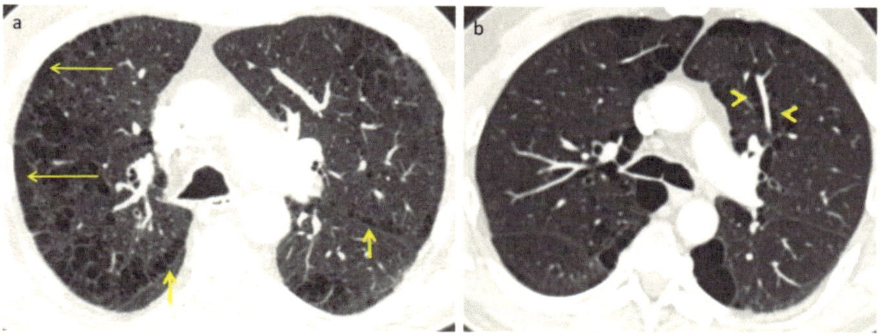

Figure 3.
(a) Seventy three year-old male with paraseptal emphysema. Axial CT images show subpleural (long arrows) and parafissural (short arrows) distribution of the emphysematous spaces demarcated by thin interlobular septa. (b) Different patient, 57 year-old male with paraseptal emphysema involving peri-bronchovascular interstitium (arrowheads).

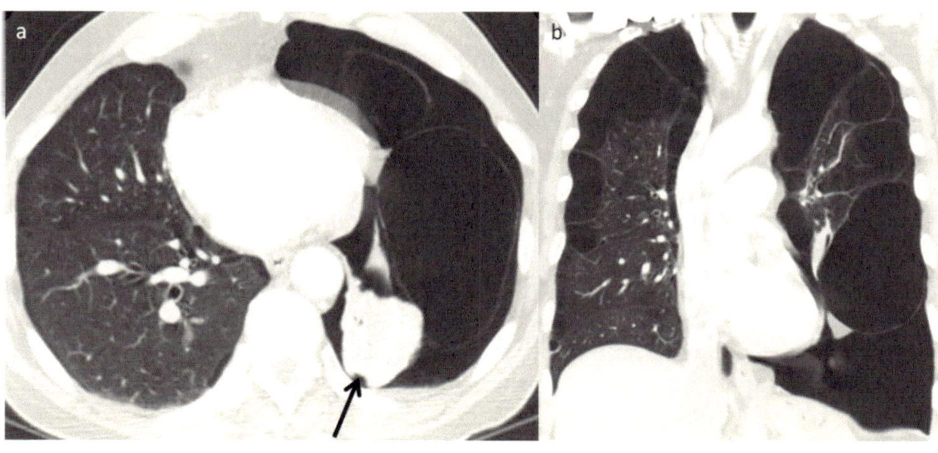

Figure 4.
Forty one year-old male with vanishing lung syndrome and recurrent pneumothorax presenting with sudden onset shortness of breath. Axial (a) and coronal (b) images of a CT demonstrated left basilar pneumothorax and large bullae, greater in the left lung. Note collapsed left lower lobe simulating a mass (arrow in a). The bullae in the left upper lobe occupy more than one third of the hemithorax compatible with VLS.

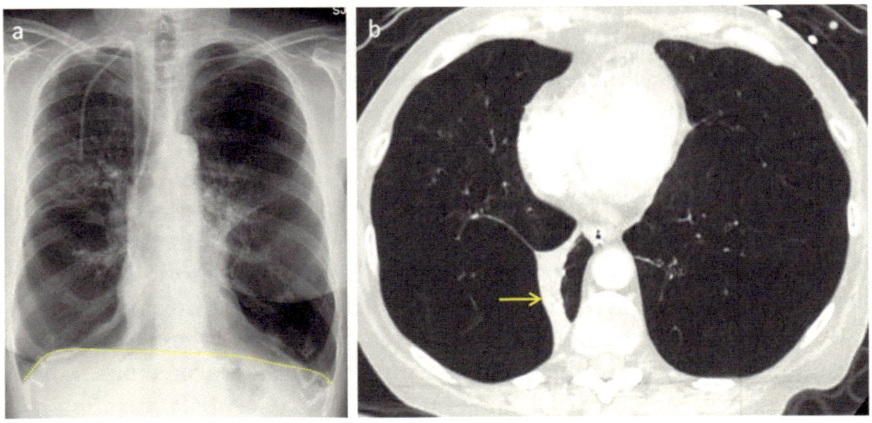

Figure 5.
Sixty four year-old female with alpha-1 antitrypsin deficiency and classical radiographic manifestations of panlobular emphysema. (a) PA CXR shows markedly increased pulmonary lucency and decreased vascularity, flattening of the diaphragm (dotted line) and widening of the intercostal spaces. (b) Axial CT image demonstrates marked hyperinflation and paucity of pulmonary vessels of the bilateral lower and right middle lobes. Note atelectatic band in the right lower lobe (arrow), likely a result of compression by hyperinflated lung.

Combined pulmonary fibrosis and emphysema syndrome (CPFE) is characterized by simultaneous occurrence of emphysema and pulmonary fibrosis. The latter commonly being of usual interstitial pneumonia (UIP) – type pattern. Spirometry testing in CPFE usually demonstrates preservation of lung volumes and normal FEV1/FVC, due to the neutralizing effects of coexisting obstructive and restrictive physiologies. On the other hand, the combined effect of emphysema and fibrosis results in a severely impaired gas exchange diagnosed as low diffusion capacity of the lung for carbon monoxide (DLCO), in these patients. The exact pathogenesis of CPFE remains uncertain, however a compiled review of published cases showed that 98% of patients with CPFE were smokers or former smokers and 90% were men [6]. Although prior reports counter-intuitively demonstrated better survival in patients with CPFE than in patients with IPF alone, Ryerson et al. recently showed no difference in survival between the two groups [7].

Imaging of CPFE is characterized by upper lobe emphysema and lower lobe pulmonary fibrosis. The emphysema may be bullous, paraseptal or centrilobular [6]. The most common fibrosis pattern in CPFE is usual interstitial pneumonia (UIP), with basilar predominant reticulations, traction bronchiectasis and bronchiolectasis, and honeycombing. Non-specific interstitial pneumonia (NSIP)-type pattern, and ground glass changes suggesting RB-ILD or DIP have been reported as well [8]. Variability of the fibrosis pattern and severity in CPFE may partly explain the conflicting reports of better survival in patients with CPFE compared to IPF. Pulmonary hypertension is an important complication and cause of mortality in CPFE and can be suggested by the presence of an enlarged pulmonary trunk on imaging. Lung cancer seems to be more prevalent in patients with CPFE than in those with isolated COPD or idiopathic pulmonary fibrosis (IPF) [6].

Giant bullous emphysema/vanishing lung syndrome (VLS) is characterized radiographically by the presence of unilateral or bilateral upper lobe giant bullae occupying at least one third of the hemithorax with associated compression of adjacent normal lung [9] (**Figure 4**). It is predominantly seen in young male smokers, who present with worsening dyspnea due to progressive expansion of the bullae [10].

On chest radiographs VLS is characterized by unilateral or bilateral thin walled lucencies in the upper lobes. Adjacent band opacities may be seen and represent adjacent compressed lung. The findings on CT include variable number of bullae varying in size between 1 and 20 cm. CT also frequently shows associated paraseptal emphysema and, to a lesser extent, centrilobular emphysema [11]. Imaging can also reveal complications of VLS, such as pneumothorax resulting from ruptured bullae, infected bullae and bronchopleural fistulas [10]. It can be difficult to distinguish the displaced visceral pleural line of pneumothorax from the linear bands seen in VLS on CXR, and CT may be needed for confirmation. In symptomatic patients, bullectomy is the treatment of choice and preoperative determination of the volume of the bullae by CT can predict the degree of improvement in lung function and FEV1 following surgery [10].

Non smoking-related emphysema: In 10% of patients, causes other than smoking are believed to result in the development of emphysema [12]. As with smoking-related emphysema, these may or may not be associated with persistent airflow limitation and therefore may or may not fit the definition of COPD. The morphological pattern of emphysema in non-smokers is sometimes vague or not specified in the medical literature, which may be partly due to its limited documentation on chest radiographs. The most common causes in adults include.

Alpha 1-Antitrypsin deficiency (AAT) is an autosomal co-dominant disease characterized by reduced levels of serum alpha-1 antitrypsin. This deficiency results in unopposed neutrophil elastase action. This results in lung destruction, hepatic cirrhosis and panniculitis. Severity of the disease is variable and dependent on specific genotype. It is often detected between the age of 35 and 45. Treatment includes substitution by exogenous alpha-1 antitrypsin [12].

On imaging ATT manifests as basal predominant panlobular emphysema (**Figure 5**). Mild disease is very difficult to distinguish from normal lung on CXR or even CT. CXR demonstrates increased lucency and reduced vascularity at the lung bases and signs of hyperinflation. CT shows widespread areas of decreased attenuation without definable walls, reflecting panlobular emphysema at the bases, and normal upper lobes. Other CT findings include paucity of the vessels in the affected areas, signs of hyperinflation such as intercostal bulging of the lungs and a saber sheath trachea. Several studies also report the presence of bronchiectasis and bronchial wall thickening in affected areas of the lung, possibly due to recurrent infection [13]. Smoking can accelerate AAT progression and associated decline in lung function [12].

Connective tissue disorders. Emphysema can be seen in patients with connective tissue disorders, including Marfan, Ehler-Danlos and Cutis laxa syndromes, thought to result from a defect in elastin. In Marfan syndrome emphysema is commonly paraseptal [14] and there may be formation of apical bullae, leading to pneumothoraces (**Figure 6**) [15]. To our knowledge, there is a single report of panacinar emphysema in Ehler-Danlos [16]. Although there are several reports of emphysema in cutis laxa, the specific morphological type is not specified in these publications, but described as 'bullous' [17].

Cicatricial emphysema, also known as paracicatricial or irregular emphysema represents airspace enlargement and lung destruction regardless of the boundaries of the acinus or secondary lobule and is usually the result of adjacent areas of scarring or fibrosis in inflammatory and granulomatous processes, such as pulmonary progressive massive fibrosis [3, 18] (**Figure 7**). Since this type of emphysema is always associated with fibrosis, it does not strictly meet the criteria for the definition of COPD, and is usually not associated with obstructive physiology [3].

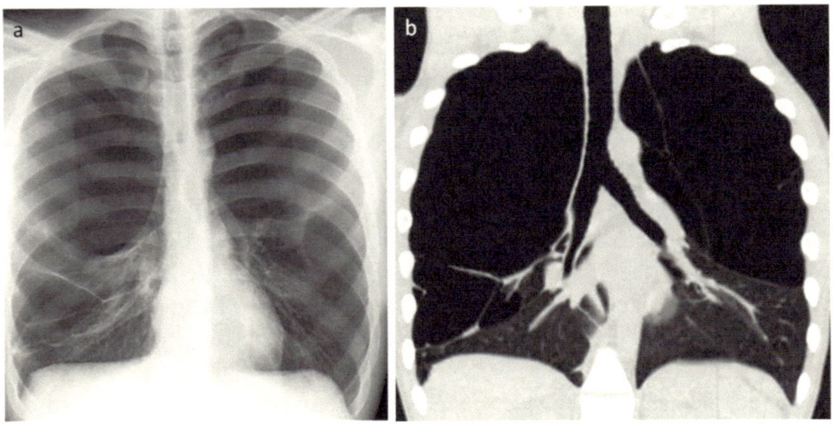

Figure 6.
Twenty eight year-old male with Marfan syndrome. (a) PA CXR shows extensive bilateral upper lung lucencies and absence of bronchovascular markings consistent with large bullae. There is compressive atelectasis, best appreciated in the right lower lung, from the mass effect of the large bullae. (b) Coronal oblique CT confirms these findings. The upper lobes are almost entirely replaced by large bullae and there is compression of the lower lungs. The patient subsequently underwent bilateral lung transplantation.

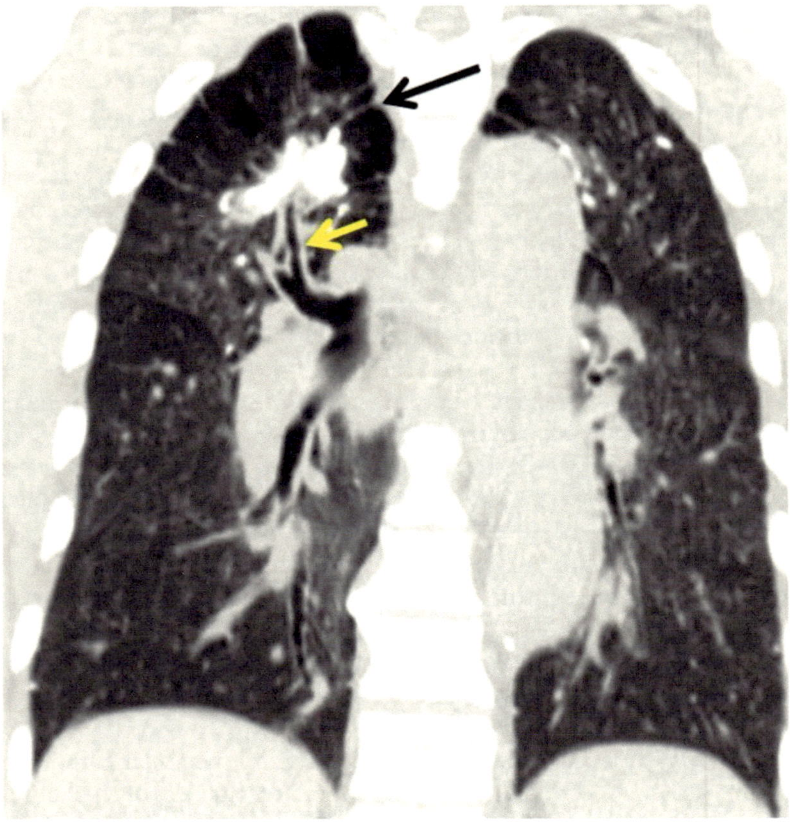

Figure 7.
Fifty six year-old male with history of crack cocaine smoking, cigarette smoking and IV drug abuse. Coronal CT image demonstrates a large calcified mass consistent with progressive massive fibrosis. There is adjacent lung destruction resulting in irregular/paracicatricial emphysema (long arrow). Note marked circumferential bronchial wall thickening (short arrow) stable for 6 years, consistent with chronic bronchitis.

Emphysema related to illicit drug abuse. Emphysema and bullous lung disease have been reported in several cases of intravenous (IV) injections of talc filler-containing drugs intended for oral administration (e.g. methylphenidate and methadone tablets), and in heroin and cocaine smokers.

In IV users of talc-containing substances, especially of methylphenidate, the emphysema pattern is panlobular, basilar and symmetric, indistinguishable for alpha-1 antitrypsin deficiency, unless associated with findings of progressive massive fibrosis in the upper lungs, related to talcosis [19, 20] (**Figure** 7).

Upper lobe bullous emphysema has been described in heroin and cocaine smokers [21, 22]. Despite being the world's most widely used illicit drug, there are only case reports describing upper lobe bullous emphysema in cannabis (marijuana) smokers [23]. In view of recent legalization of cannabis in many US states and countries, and potential increased recreational use, systematic analytical studies are needed to assess its association with emphysema.

Emphysema in HIV patients. HIV seropositivity is an independent risk factor for the development of COPD and emphysema [24]. Diaz et al. found a 15% incidence of emphysema in a cohort of HIV positive patients compared to a 2% incidence in the control HIV-negative group [24]. The mechanism is not fully understood and could be potentially the result of complex immune, apoptotic, proteolytic and oxidative stress responses causing lung destruction over time [25]. On imaging, emphysema preferentially affects the upper lobes and should not be confused with cystic lung disease seen in *Pneumocystis jirovecii* infection.

Hypocomplementemic Urticarial Vasculitis syndrome (HUVS) is a rare immune complex-mediated disorder affecting multiple organs and clinically presenting with chronic urticaria, angioedema, arthritis or synovitis, conjunctivitis, uveitis, renal insufficiency and abdominal pain. It is 8 times more common in women, usually peaks in the 5th decade of life and may be associated with systemic lupus. Diagnosis is made by skin biopsy showing leukocytoclastic vasculitis and/or presence of anti-C1q antibodies in serum. HUVS may result in panlobular basilar emphysema indistinguishable from that of alpha-1 antitrypsin deficiency. Lung involvement is an important cause of morbidity and mortality in HUVS patients [26].

3. Radiography

Chest radiography plays a frontline role in the assessment of COPD and COPD exacerbations. It has the advantage of being a fast and easy exam to perform in various settings, requires minimal cooperation from patients, has minimal radiation exposure and is inexpensive.

The radiographic signs of emphysema and accuracy of its diagnosis by chest radiography were comprehensively assessed in the classic study by Thurlbeck and Simon [27], who correlated pathological findings of emphysema in 696 necropsies with ante mortem radiographs and pulmonary function test data. The salient findings of this study were five-fold. (1). The diagnostic accuracy of emphysema is highly dependent on the severity of the disease: the frequency of accurate radiological diagnosis was less than 5% in mild disease, 12–20% in moderate disease, and 50%–67% in cases of severe emphysema. (2). Corroborative clinical history (e.g. known alpha-1 antitrypsin deficiency or history of unilateral lung transplant) increases diagnostic accuracy. (3). Panacinar emphysema is more likely to be diagnosed radiographically than other types of emphysema (**Figure** 5). (4). Superimposed acute or chronic lung disease might obscure the typical radiographic findings of emphysema: the frequency of accurate diagnosis of emphysema dropped from 67 to 41% in patients with a superimposed active lung disease and (5). Quantitative radiographic assessment of emphysema is of little benefit and in clinical practice the diagnosis of emphysema on chest radiograph remains qualitative and highly subjective. The interpretation of findings is prone to inter-observer and intra-observer variability.

The radiographic features of emphysema reflect the presence of parenchymal destruction, vascular remodeling and hyperinflation (**Table 2**). These comprise the following:

Bullae are the result of coalescing emphysematous spaces, 1 cm or more in diameter [28]. They are the only direct sign of emphysema, sometimes seen on chest radiographs but better appreciated on CT. Bullae appear as well-demarcated areas of increased lucency, devoid of lung markings (**Figure 6**).

Increased radiolucency of the lungs is the result of small, scattered emphysematous spaces and constitutes an indirect sign of lung destruction (**Figures 1, 5, 6,** and **8**).

Vascular attenuation is present when there is paucity or absence of vessels in the outer third of the lung (**Figures 1, 5,** and **9**). Vessels may be completely absent secondary to bullae or in severe emphysema, or they can be present but narrowed or impoverished ("pruning"). The causes of this phenomenon may include passive compression of small vessels in the lung periphery by emphysematous spaces, hypoxic vasoconstriction and/or vascular remodeling [29].

Hyperinflation results from air-trapping and bullous formation, and manifests itself radiographically as diaphragmatic flattening, increased retrosternal space and antero-posterior (AP) diameter of the chest on lateral radiographs ("barrel chest"), widened intercostal spaces and narrowed cardiac silhouette on frontal radiographs (**Figures 1** and **9**).

Saber sheath trachea refers to the radiographic appearance of the trachea when its sagittal-to-coronal diameters ratio is greater than 2. This tracheal configuration is

Signs of parenchymal destruction and vascular remodeling
→Bullae
→Increased radiolucency of the lungs
→Vascular attenuation or complete absence of vasculature
Signs of hyperinflation and air trapping
→Flattening of the diaphragm
→Increased retrosternal space
→Increased AP diameter of the chest
→Widened intercostal spaces
→Narrowed cardiac silhouette
Supportive signs
→Saber sheath trachea
→Increased lung markings

Table 2.
Radiographic features of emphysema.

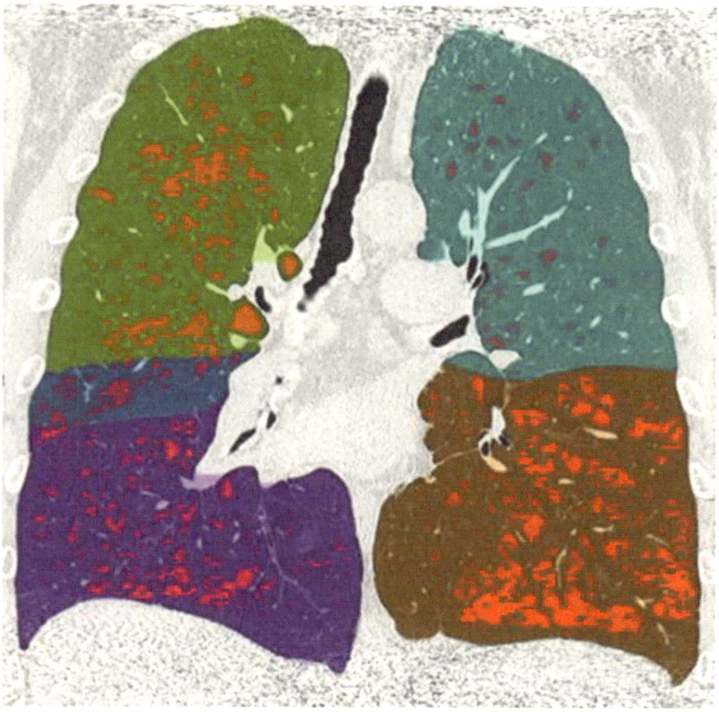

Figure 8.
Sixty seven year-old male, ex-smoker with 100 pack-years smoking history, with centrilobular emphysema and COPD. Coronal CT demonstrate COPD quantification using commercially available software (Philips IntelliSpace portal, Philips healthcare V8.0). Using a threshold of −950 HU it shows centrilobular emphysema present in all lobes (red color). Volumetric measurements and emphysema ratios are obtained for both lungs and all lobes. The emphysema ratio for both lungs is 8.5%. Emphysema is worst in the right upper lobe (emphysema ratio 11.3%).

highly associated with obstructive airway disease [30]. It may be the result of chronic airflow limitation during expiration [31].

Increased lung markings also referred to as "dirty lungs" are the result of chronic bronchitis, which is often concomitant with emphysema.

When considered separately, each of the above radiographic features has low specificity and sensitivity for diagnosis of emphysema. However, co-occurrence of several of these findings allows detection of most cases of moderate and severe emphysema and some cases of mild emphysema [32]. In a study by Sutinen et al., the combined findings of hyperinflation and vascular alterations allowed accurate diagnosis of emphysema in 97% symptomatic and in 47% of asymptomatic subjects with necropsy-proven emphysema [33].

4. Computed tomography (CT)

CT is superior to chest radiography in detection of emphysema. Similarly, disease progression is much easier to detect on CT than on chest radiography. CT also provides superior information regarding distribution and extent of the disease, which might allow determination of the cause of emphysema and its subtype.

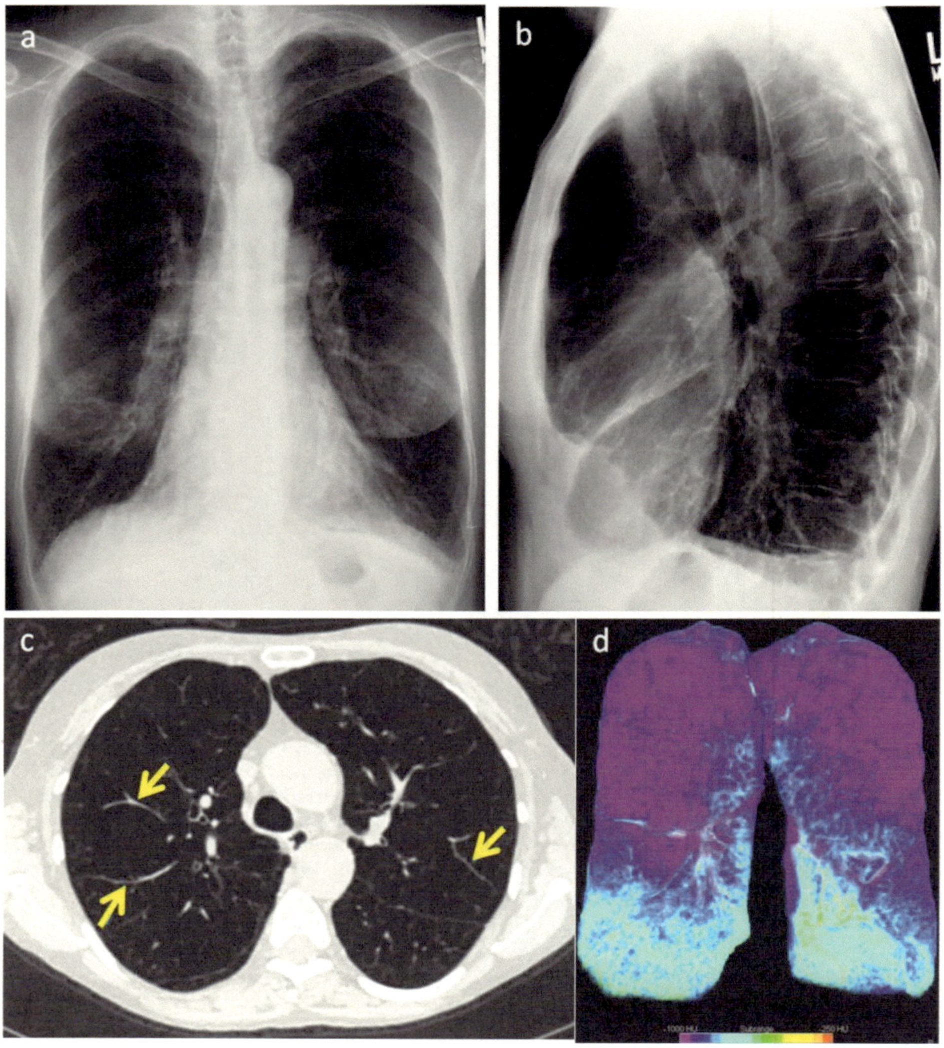

Figure 9.
Fifty year-old female with end-stage COPD, undergoing pre-transplant assessment. (a) frontal CXR shows increased radiolucency and vascular attenuation/irregularity especially in the upper lungs, widened intercostal spaces and elongation of the cardiac silhouette. (b) Lateral CXR shows increased retrosternal space, increased AP diameter of the chest and flattening of the hemidiaphragms. Notice enlarged pulmonary artery in this patient with associated pulmonary hypertension. (c) axial CT image confirms marked increased radiolucency (−990 HU in the right upper lobe) and vascular irregularity (arrows) predominating in the upper lungs, compatible with severe emphysema. Coronal (30° caudal angulation) CT ventilation map (d) showing abnormally low attenuation values in the upper lungs (close to -1000HU) compatible with severe emphysema. The patient subsequently underwent double lung transplantation.

Emphysema can be readily detected on conventional CT with 5–10 mm slice thickness, however is best depicted with high-resolution CT with 1–2 mm slice thickness reconstructed with a lung algorithm [34]. Using modern multislice CT scanners, such acquisitions can be obtained at full inspiration during a single breath-hold. Coronal and sagittal reformations are helpful in assessment of the distribution and extent of emphysema. Although intravenous contrast is not required for the assessment of emphysema, pulmonary blood volume imaging obtained from dual energy CT (a computed tomography technique that uses two separate x-ray photon energy spectra,

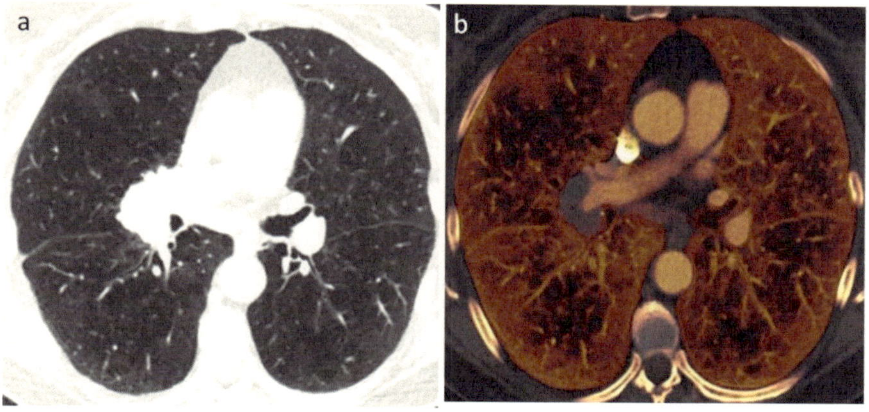

Figure 10.
Seventy nine year-old female with a 50 pack-year history of smoking. Axial CT (a) and corresponding pulmonary blood volume image (b) at midlung level show decreased perfusion in areas of emphysema.

allowing the interrogation of materials that have different attenuation properties at different energies) may aid in the detection of emphysema by highlighting areas of hypo-perfusion (**Figure 10**).

On CT, emphysema appears as focal, regional, or diffuse areas of low attenuation, contrasting with surrounding normal lung. In addition, all conventional radiographic features of emphysema, such as the attenuation of the caliber of the vessels in emphysematous regions, may be identified on CT. Features of hyperinflation may be better appreciated on coronal and sagittal reformations than on axial images. The severity of emphysema in various regions of the lungs can be visually and subjectively estimated by scrolling though all available CT images in any plane and rating them on a four point scale as (1) < 25% of the area (2) 26%–50% of the area, (3) 51%–75% of the area, or (4) > 75% of the area [31].

When correlated with histopathology (gold standard), the accuracy of CT for both, detection of emphysema and of its distribution, increases with thin collimation high-resolution computed tomography (HRCT) [35]. When correlated with the pathologic grade of emphysema, HRCT performance is excellent in vitro (r = 0.91), and slightly lower but strong-to-very strong in vivo (r = 0.7–0.9), although very mild emphysema may be missed [32].

CT is more sensitive than pulmonary function tests for the detection of emphysema. In a study involving 615 men ranging in age from 40 to 69 years, who underwent lung cancer screening with low-dose spiral CT, emphysema was detected in 30% of current smokers (116/380); of these, the majority had normal spirometry results (78%). Additional studies have also shown that 68–80% of smokers with emphysema detected on HRCT had normal spirometry results [35].

The sensitivity for detection of subtle emphysema can be improved by using the MinIP (minimum intensity projection) technique [36]. Contrary to the MIP (maximum intensity projection), which is helpful in the detection of high attenuation structures such as vessels and lung nodules, the MinIP technique recognizes the regions of the lung with the lowest attenuation values such as emphysema, while subtracting the normal lung and pulmonary vasculature. This technique is however not widely used in clinical practice due the extra steps involved in producing these images and their limited clinical value.

5. Quantitative assessment of emphysema

The two main techniques used to quantify the extent of emphysema on CT are the threshold technique and histogram analysis. These are based on the simple fact that emphysematous lung has lower attenuation than normal lung parenchyma. Since the introduction of these techniques several variations have been introduced, mainly as a result of improvements in CT capabilities and image processing software. Such examples include 3D assessment of whole lung density, made possible by fast image acquisition of the entire lung volume using multidetector CT.

Threshold technique. In this technique, emphysema is considered to be present if the attenuation value of the pixels in the area of interest falls below an absolute predetermined Hounsfield unit threshold value [37]. The threshold value of – 950HU for detection of emphysema has been shown to correlate well with pulmonary function tests and pathological data when using thin section CT at 10 mm interval (**Figure 8**) [38, 39]. (For reference, the value of −1000 HU corresponds to radiodensity air and 0 HU to that of water.) Prior to that, Muller et al. had used a software program called density mask to highlight voxels falling within a predetermined range, and found that a threshold value of −910 HU correlated best with the extent of emphysema when using a 10 mm slice thickness [40]. The use of other threshold values, ranging between −900 and −980 HU, has also been reported and is dependent on a variety of factors including scanning parameters [37].

Histogram analysis. In this technique, emphysema is detected if the attenuation value of a pixel falls below a predetermined percentile. The enlargement of the air spaces distal to the terminal bronchioles, accompanied by destruction of alveolar walls in emphysema, results in a reduced ratio of the surface area of the walls of distal airspaces per unit lung volume (AWUV) [41]. In their CT-pathologic correlation study, Gould et al. showed significant correlation between AWUV and the lowest 5th percentile of the CT density histogram ($r = -0.77$) [41]. Contrary to the threshold technique, where an absolute number is predetermined as an indicator of emphysema, histogram analysis can underestimate the extent of emphysema if a concomitant disease (such as pulmonary mass or consolidation) shifts the histogram curve towards higher overall Hounsfield values [34].

6. Imaging of comorbidities associated with COPD

Imaging is also valuable in establishing the presence of co-morbidities frequently associated with COPD. The most common association is with heart failure and ischemic heart disease. Emphysema can also eventually lead to pulmonary hypertension and right heart failure with radiographs and CT showing enlarged central pulmonary arteries and cardiomegaly. Pulmonary hypertension has been estimated to be present in 35 to 90% of patients with COPD and its presence is associated with greater mortality and morbidity [42].

Lung cancer is the most frequent cause of death in patients with mild to moderate COPD, whereas infections are the most common cause of COPD exacerbations and are associated with significant mortality [1].

The radiologist should therefore look for and report signs suggestive of these comorbidities, such as coronary and aortic atherosclerosis, cardiomegaly, enlarged pulmonary arteries, pulmonary edema, pleural effusions, pulmonary nodules, masses and consolidations.

7. Conclusion

Radiological imaging modalities, such as radiography and CT, are crucial in diagnosis and quantification of emphysema, in differentiating among its different subtypes and identification of its potential etiologies, monitoring of disease and complications, and management of these entities. Newer techniques in quantitative CT can provide more objective, reproducible and more reliable longitudinal assessment of emphysema, however these techniques need to be validated in large cohorts and their current use remains limited in clinical practice.

Conflict of interest

The authors declare no conflict of interest.

Author details

Karl Sayegh[1], Josephine Pressacco[2], Bojan Kovacina[3], Subba Digumarthy[4] and Alexandre Semionov[2]*

1 Department of Radiology, Baptist Health South Florida, Miami, Florida, USA

2 Department of Radiology, McGill University Health Center, Montreal, Canada

3 Department of Radiology, Jewish General Hospital, Montreal, Canada

4 Department of Radiology, Massachusetts General Hospital, Boston, USA

*Address all correspondence to: alexandre.semionov@mail.mcgill.ca

References

[1] Vestbo J, Hurd SS, Agustí AG, Jones PW, Vogelmeier C, Anzueto A, et al. Global strategy for the diagnosis, management, and prevention of chronic obstructive pulmonary disease. American Journal of Respiratory and Critical Care Medicine. 2013;**187**(4):347-365. DOI: 10.1164/rccm.201204-0596PP

[2] Snider G, Klinerman J, Thurlbeck WM. The definition of emphysema: Report of the National Heart, Lung, and Blood Institute division of lung diseases workshop. The American Review of Respiratory Disease. 1985;**132**:182-185

[3] Stern EJ, Frank MS. CT of the lung in patients with pulmonary emphysema: Diagnosis, quantification, and correlation with pathologic and physiologic findings. American Journal of Roentgenology. 1994;**162**(4):791-798. DOI: 10.2214/ajr.162.4.8140992

[4] Takahashi M, Fukuoka J, Nitta N, Takazakura R, Nagatani Y, Murakami Y, et al. Imaging of pulmonary emphysema: A pictorial review. International Journal of Chronic Obstructive Pulmonary Disease. 2008;**3**(2):193

[5] Naidich DP, McCauley DI, Khouri NF, et al. Computed tomography of bronchiectasis. Journal of Computer Assisted Tomography. 1982;**6**:437-444

[6] Jankowich MD. Combined pulmonary fibrosis and emphysema syndrome. Chest Journal. 2012;**141**(1):1-10. DOI: 10.1378/chest.11-1062

[7] Ryerson CJ, Hartman T, Elicker BM, Ley B, Lee JS, Abbritti M, et al. Clinical features and outcomes in combined pulmonary fibrosis and emphysema in idiopathic pulmonary fibrosis. Chest Journal. 2013;**144**(1):234. DOI: 10.1378/chest.12-2403

[8] Attili AK, Kazerooni EA, Gross BH, Flaherty KR, Myers JL, Martinez FJ. Smoking-related interstitial lung disease: Radiologic-clinical-pathologic correlation. Radiographics. 2008;**28**(5):1383-1396

[9] Roberts L, Putman CE, Chen JTT, et al. Vanishing lung syndrome: Upper lobe bullous pneumopathy. Revista Interamericana de Radiología. 1987;**12**:249-255

[10] Sharma N, Justaniah AM, Kanne JP, Gurney JW, Mohammed T-LH. Vanishing lung syndrome (giant bullous emphysema): CT findings in 7 patients and a literature review. Journal of Thoracic Imaging. 2009;**24**(3):227-230. DOI: 10.1097/RTI.0b013e31819b9f2a

[11] Stern EJ, Webb WR, Weinacker A, Müller NL. Idiopathic giant bullous emphysema (vanishing lung syndrome): Imaging findings in nine patients. American Journal of Roentgenology. 1994;**162**(2):279-282. DOI: 10.2214/ajr.162.2.8310909

[12] Lee P, Gildea TR, Stoller JK. Emphysema in nonsmokers: Alpha 1-antitrypsin deficiency and other causes. Cleveland Clinic Journal of Medicine. 2002;**69**(12):928-936

[13] Shaker SB, Stavngaard T, Stolk J, Stoel B, Dirksen A. Alpha1-antitrypsin deficiency. 7: Computed tomographic imaging in alpha1-antitrypsin deficiency. Thorax. 2004;**59**(11):986-991. DOI: 10.1136/thorax.2003.006569

[14] Dyhdalo K, Farver C. Pulmonary histologic changes in Marfan syndrome:

A case series and literature review. American Journal of Clinical Pathology. 2011;**136**(6):857-863

[15] Wood JR, Bellamy D, Child AH, Citron KM. Pulmonary disease in patients with Marfan syndrome. Thorax. 1984;**39**(10):780-784

[16] Cupo LN, Pyeritz RE, Olson JL, McPhee SJ, Hutchins GM, McKusick VA. Ehlers-Danlos syndrome with abnormal collagen fibrils, sinus of Valsalva aneurysms, myocardial infarction, panacinar emphysema and cerebral heterotopias. The American Journal of Medicine. 1981;**71**(6):1051-1058. DOI: 10.1016/0002-9343(81)90341-7

[17] Turner-Stokes L, Turton C, Pope FM, Green M. Emphysema and cutis laxa. Thorax. 1983;**38**(10):790-792

[18] Foster WL, Gimenez EI, Roubidoux MA, Sherrier RH, Shannon RH, Roggli VL, et al. The emphysemas: Radiologic-pathologic correlations. Radiographics: A Review Publication of the Radiological Society of North America, Inc. 1993;**13**(2):311-328

[19] Stern EJ, Frank MS, Schmutz JF, Glenny RW, Schmidt RA, Godwin JD. Panlobular pulmonary emphysema caused by i.v. injection of methylphenidate (Ritalin): Findings on chest radiographs and CT scans. American Journal of Roentgenology. 1994;**162**(3):555-560. DOI: 10.2214/ajr.162.3.8109495

[20] Ward S, Heyneman LE, Reittner P, Kazerooni EA, Godwin JD, Müller NL. Talcosis associated with IV abuse of oral medications: CT findings. American Journal of Roentgenology. 2000;**174**(3):789-793. DOI: 10.2214/ajr.174.3.1740789

[21] Van der Klooster JM, Grootendorst AF. Severe bullous emphysema associated with cocaine smoking. Thorax. 2001;**56**(12):982-983

[22] Walker PP, Thwaite E, Amin S, Curtis JM, Calverley PMA. The association between heroin inhalation and early onset emphysema. Chest. 2015;**148**(5):1156-1163. DOI: 10.1378/chest.15-0236

[23] Johnson MR, Smith RP, Morrison D, et al. Large lung bullae in marijuana smokers. Thorax. 2000;**55**:340-342

[24] Diaz PT, King MA, Pacht ER, Wewers MD, Gadek JE, Nagaraja HN, et al. Increased susceptibility to pulmonary emphysema among HIV-seropositive smokers. Annals of Internal Medicine. 2000;**132**(5):369-372

[25] Petrache I, Diab K, Knox KS, Twigg HL, Stephens RS, Flores S, et al. HIV associated pulmonary emphysema: A review of the literature and inquiry into its mechanism. Thorax. 2008;**63**(5):463-469. DOI: 10.1136/thx.2007.079111

[26] Pujara AC, Mohammed T-LH. Hypocomplementemic urticarial vasculitis syndrome: A rare cause of basilar panacinar emphysema. Journal of Thoracic Imaging. 2012;**27**(3):W50-W51. DOI: 10.1097/RTI.0b013e31822770fb

[27] Thurlbeck WM, Simon G. Radiographic appearance of the chest in emphysema. American Journal of Roentgenology. 1978;**130**(3):429-440. DOI: 10.2214/ajr.130.3.429

[28] Hansell DM, Bankier AA, MacMahon H, McLoud TC, Müller NL, Remy J. Fleischner society: Glossary of terms for thoracic imaging. Radiology. 2008;**246**(3):697-722. DOI: 10.1148/radiol.2462070712

[29] Matsuoka S, Yamashiro T, Washko GR, Kurihara Y, Nakajima Y, Hatabu H. Quantitative ct assessment of chronic obstructive pulmonary disease 1. Radiographics: A Review Publication of the Radiological Society of North America, Inc. 2010;**30**(1):55-66

[30] Greene R, Lechner GL. "Saber-sheath" trachea: A clinical and functional study of marked coronal narrowing of the intrathoracic trachea. Radiology. 1975;**115**:265-268

[31] Friedman PJ. Imaging studies in emphysema. Proceedings of the American Thoracic Society. 2008;**5**(4):494-500. DOI: 10.1513/pats.200708-128ET

[32] Muller N, Coxson H. Chronic obstructive pulmonary disease 4: Imaging the lungs in patients with chronic obstructive pulmonary disease. Thorax. 2002;**57**(11):982

[33] Sutinen S, Christoforidis AJ, Klugh GA, et al. Roentgenologic criteria for the recognition of nonsymptomatic pulmonary emphysema: Correlation between roentgenologic findings and pulmonary pathology. The American Review of Respiratory Disease. 1965;**91**:69-76

[34] Litmanovich D, Boiselle PM, Bankier AA. CT of pulmonary emphysema - Current status, challenges, and future directions. European Radiology. 2008;**19**(3):537-551. DOI: 10.1007/s00330-008-1186-4

[35] Omori H, Nakashima R, Otsuka N, Mishima Y, Tomiguchi S, Narimatsu A, et al. Emphysema detected by lung cancer screening with low-dose spiral CT: Prevalence, and correlation with smoking habits and pulmonary function in Japanese male subjects. Respirology (Carlton Vic). 2006;**11**(2):205-210. DOI: 10.1111/j.1440-1843.2006.00827

[36] Remy-Jardin M, Remy J, Gosselin B, et al. Sliding thin slab, minimumintensity projection technique in the diagnosis of emphysema: Histopathologic-CT correlation. Radiology. 1996;**200**:665-671

[37] Newell JD. Quantitative computed tomography of lung parenchyma in chronic obstructive pulmonary disease: An overview. Proceedings of the American Thoracic Society. 2008;**5**(9):915-918. DOI: 10.1513/pats.200804-034QC

[38] Gevenois PA, de Maertelaer V, De Vuyst P, et al. Comparison of computed density and macroscopic morphometry in pulmonary emphysema. American Journal of Respiratory and Critical Care Medicine. 1995;**152**:653-657

[39] Gevenois PA, De Vuyst P, de Maertelaer V, et al. Comparison of computed density and microscopic morphometry in pulmonary emphysema. American Journal of Respiratory and Critical Care Medicine. 1996;**154**:187-192

[40] Müller NL, Staples CA, Miller RR, et al. "Density mask": An objective method to quantitate emphysema using computed tomography. Chest. 1988;**94**:782-787

[41] Gould GAG, MacNee WW, McLean AA, Warren PMP, Redpath AA, Best JJJ, et al. CT measurements of lung density in life can quantitate distal airspace enlargement - An essential defining feature of human emphysema. The American Review of Respiratory Disease. 1988;**137**(2):380-392

[42] Washko G. Diagnostic Imaging in COPD. Seminars in Respiratory and Critical Care Medicine. 2010;**31**(03):276-285. DOI: 10.1055/s-0030-1254068

Section 4

Consequences

Chapter 5

Influence of Chronic Obstructive Pulmonary Disease on Work Ability

Jasmina Biscevic-Tokic, Zurifa Ajanovic, Sanja Brekalo-Lazarevic and Nedim Tokic

Abstract

Chronic obstructive pulmonary disease (COPD) is a leading cause of mortality, morbidity and disability worldwide. COPD cannot always be defined as an occupational disease, because it is more of a work-related disease or a disease that worsens at work, and the patient's ability to work will depend on the degree and duration of lung function damage. Very clearly and unambiguously, apart from smoking as a risk factor for the development of COPD, the workplace and work environment are also important. In our research, the largest number of patients with COPD worked at workplaces with special working conditions and were exposed to chemical, physical, and biological hazards at the workplace, which brings with it an increased number of sick days due to frequent exacerbations of the disease and reduced work ability.

Keywords: workplace and environment, work capacity, chronic obstructive pulmonary disease, work-related illness, prevention

1. Introduction

Cigarette smoking is the best-known and most common cause of chronic obstructive pulmonary disease (COPD) in the world [1]. Cigarette smoke causes airway inflammation in COPD, which is known to persist even after smoking cessation [2]. Other causes are more common in developing countries, namely passive smoking, environmental and workplace exposure, and lack of alpha-1-antitrypsin.

Indoor and outdoor air pollution is an important cause of the onset and development of COPD [3]. Certain professions where patients are exposed to harmful particles and gases at the workplace also represent risk factors for the onset of disease [4].

Given that chronic obstructive pulmonary disease is a multicomponent disease that, due to symptoms, therapy, and changes in functionality, leads to altered work ability and more frequent sick days, with our study we wanted to draw attention to how important the workplace of workers, especially in industry, contributes to the initiation of the disease and exposure to risks that may further exacerbate it.

COPD cannot always be defined as an occupational disease, as it is more of a work-related disease or a disease aggravated by work along with smoking. Many epidemiological studies have confirmed that long-term occupational exposure to various dusts increases the risk of developing COPD [5].

For work processes in which there is exposure to gases, vapors, and dusts, as well as unfavorable microclimatic conditions, the risk of exposure as well as the length of exposure at the workplace must be assessed. When it comes to dusts, the most common occupations for an increased risk of COPD are in the production of ceramics, barite cement, lignite, and brown coal mines. These are dusts with a possible fibrogenic effect, and relatively inert dusts. In technical and technological processes in production, there are numerous toxic substances that serve as raw materials. The synergy of several raw materials in the process of obtaining a finished final product is worse than a finished chemical compound. Inhalation of such compounds acts as one of the factors for exacerbation of COPD or, during prolonged exposure, for the development of the disease [6].

The evaluation of working capacity will depend on the degree and durability of lung function damage, so we evaluate it in the following way:

- Slight impairment of lung function (FEV1 > 80%), does not reduce the ability to work for the largest number of occupations.

- Moderate impairment of lung function (30% > FEV1 < 80%) leads to inability to work with moderate and severe physical exertion.

- Severe pulmonary function impairment (FEV1 < 30%) prevents any physical effort.

The measurement of the partial pressures of oxygen and carbon dioxide is also of great importance for the assessment of work capacity [7].

The ventilation of the space where the worker resides is important because synergistic action is also possible in the atmosphere of the present pollution.

Every worker suffering from COPD requires a change of workplace when the presence of respiratory irritants is found at the workplace, even when they do not exceed the maximum permissible concentration (MDK) [8].

At least every 2 years, they must undergo health examinations, which must include a diagnostic minimum for exposure to gases, vapors and dusts. The life of patients with COPD can be stressful because it forces life changes, which are also reflected in work functioning [9].

COPD is significant not only due to its large spread, but also due to economic pressure on health insurance funds, where large funds are allocated for the treatment and rehabilitation of patients [10, 11]. According to data from the World Health Organization (WHO), COPD is the fourth leading cause of death, after cardiovascular, malignant and cerebrovascular diseases. Nowadays, there is a significant increase in costs for the treatment of chronic lung diseases in the total costs of health care. The more severe the chronic disease, according to the Global Initiative for Chronic Obstructive Lung Disease (GOLD) [12], the higher the direct and indirect costs of treatment [13]. Indirect costs include loss of working ability, absence from work – sick leave, patient care and others. Indirect costs can be classified into two types: morbidity costs (time lost from work due to illness) and mortality costs (time lost due to premature death) [14].

The costs of sick leave, loss of working ability of patients with respiratory diseases, are estimated to amount to 41.4 billion euros, and COPD is responsible for more than half of this amount, i.e. 25.1 billion euros [15]. Since human capital is often the most important national asset for developing countries, the indirect costs of COPD could be a serious threat to their economies. This group of patients should be the focus of attention of workers, employers, and doctors, as well as health and pension insurance agencies [16, 17].

Men tend to have exacerbations more often, but in recent years the difference has decreased due to the increase in the number of smokers among women . The study conducted by Ljubičić [18] included 61 subjects with COPD, of which 41 (67.2%) were male and 20 (32.8%) were female. Such results may arise because male respondents mostly work at workplaces with special working conditions and are exposed to harmful noxious agents from both the workplace and the environment.

According to data published so far, approximately 328 million people suffer from COPD worldwide, of which 168 million are men and 160 million are women [18]. COPD usually occurs after the age of 40 and is mostly related to long-term smoking, although exposure to harmful workplace and environmental factors cannot be ruled out.

The GOLD report [12] describes the ABCD test, which divides COPD patients into four groups, A, B, C, and D. Groups A and B are low risk and have zero to one exacerbations per year, not leading to hospital admission, where Group A has less symptoms and Group B has more symptoms. Groups C and D are high risk and have two or more exacerbations or one or more hospitalizations per year, with Group C having less symptoms and Group D having more symptoms.

2. Material and methods

During the examination in 2019 in the Pulmonology Cabinet of the Health Center, a prospective study was conducted using appropriate questionnaires with a smaller retrospective part using previous medical documentation (medical history and other medical documentation), which included 150 respondents (workers) with already established and verified diagnosis of COPD. In the examined group, subgroups were formed in relation to the habit of consuming cigarettes (smokers and non-smokers), as one of the most important risk factors for the development of COPD.

Criteria for inclusion in the study:

- Patients older than 40 years.
- Diagnosed with chronic obstructive pulmonary disease.
- Voluntary consent to participate in research.

Criteria for exclusion from the study:

- Patients under 40 years of age.
- Workers suffering from malignant diseases and pneumoconiosis.
- That they do not suffer from COPD.
- To have no other comorbidities.
- Without voluntary consent to participate in research.

Each worker was examined by an occupational medicine specialist who performed and interpreted additional tests.

1. A detailed anamnesis was taken for each subject with a special emphasis on the work anamnesis, absence from work and the habit of consuming cigarettes.

2. Each subject filled out a standardized questionnaire for COPD (CAT questionnaire).

   The COPD assessment test (CAT) questionnaire was created as a result of the need for doctors to better understand their patients' condition in order to achieve the optimal treatment of COPD. The description of the disease, which was taken as the framework concept of the questionnaire, was created after numerous expert meetings with doctors and patients. Additionally, two validation studies as well as patient testing were performed as part of the European Quality of Life Survey. The entire research resulted in a short, simple, validated questionnaire consisting of eight simple questions that provide the best framework concept for the description of the disease. Each question quantifies the impact of the disease on the patient's quality of life based on a semantic scale from zero to five. The values on this scale are circled by the patient for each of the eight questions. The values of the obtained results range from 0 to 40. While spirometry remains the gold standard for confirming the diagnosis and determining the severity and stage of COPD, but it does not fully reflect the impact of this disease on patients' lives.

3. A physical examination was performed with special emphasis on auscultatory findings on the lungs.

4. Anthropometric measurements were taken, including body mass (BW), body height (BW).

   An anthropometer according to Martin was used to measure body height (BH) with a measurement accuracy of 0.1 cm. Each subject was measured without shoes, hands relaxed next to the body, heels together, with the head positioned so that the so-called the Frankfurt plane (an imaginary line connecting the tragus of the auricle and the outer corner of the eye) should be horizontal.
   A medical decimal scale with a movable weight was used to measure body mass. The measurement accuracy on the same is +/−0.3 kg.
   The spirometric examination was performed in the Pulmonology Office of the Sarajevo Hospital on the "Master Screen Body Jaeger" spirometer, which was manufactured in Germany.

5. Spirometry is the gold standard for diagnosing chronic obstructive pulmonary disease (COPD). It is a simple, quick and painless test that is performed to assess lung function by measuring the volume of air that the patient can exhale from the lungs after maximal exhalation. The patient was explained how to test the lung function and how he should cooperate with the nurse in order for the findings to be technically correct. The patient's nose must be plugged with a clip. The patient will first breathe normally through the mouthpiece, which he has covered well with his lips.

   The patient then breathes with forced inhalation and exhalation. This respiration was repeated three times, and the best result will be taken for analysis.

Lung volumes (respiratory volume, inspiratory reserve volume, expiratory reserve volume) and capacities (vital capacity, inspiratory capacity), as well as respiratory volumes as a function of time (forced expiratory volumes) are determined by spirometric testing. During the forced expiratory maneuver, vital capacity is obtained, which in this case is marked as forced vital capacity (FVC) and forced expiratory volume during the first second (FEV1) as well as flow rates in the flow/volume curve.

6. We monitored working capacity on the basis of absence from work and monitoring of spirometric findings.

3. Results

The study that we conducted confirmed that COPD significantly affects the working ability of the respondents, and therefore the quality of life in all its spheres. The study included 150 subjects suffering from COPD, 105 male subjects and 45 female subjects.

Our study, compared to others, included more male patients with irreversible airway obstruction. The average age of our subjects was 60.16 years (SD ± 5.12 years) (**Table 1**).

Most of the respondents who had chronic obstructive pulmonary disease were from the 60 to 70 age group (55.00%). This was expected because COPD takes decades to fully develop. The group up to 70 years of age was taken into the research because employees in certain workplaces had the possibility to work up to 70 years of age. In the research of Skrbić, the average age of the subjects was 64.85 years ±10.1, which is a similar value as in our research [19]. Therefore, the higher the age, the greater the number of people with COPD, which brings with it an increased number of sick days due to frequent exacerbations of the disease and reduced work capacity.

The analysis of the COPD stage of the subjects of this study, according to the GOLD ABCD tool, yielded the results reported in **Table 2**. Most respondents were in the group with moderately severe and severe stage of the disease. In these patients, due to their age, especially if they have not stopped smoking, the disease is expected to worsen, with occasional hospitalizations, due to progressing symptoms. COPD worsens progressively, and it is often difficult to find the cause of the exacerbation of the disease and the transition to a more severe stage. The results of our study agree with results of the study of Maričić. and most respondents were in the group with stages B and C [20]. According to data from the Institute of Public Health of the Federation of Bosnia and Herzegovina, it is believed that one in 10 inhabitants of Europe has a mild or severe form of COPD, and that the large number of smokers among the inhabitants of the Federation of Bosnia and Herzegovina (44.1%), as well as increasing air pollution affects are major contributors to the causes of death [21].

Minimum age	Maximum age	Average age of respondents	The age range is	Standard deviation SD
40 years	70 years	60.16 years	30 years	±5.12 years

Table 1.
Demographic characteristics of subjects with COPD (age).

COPD stage	Number of patients	Percentage in relation to the total number of patients
A	33	22.00%
B	40	26.67%
C	44	29.33%
D	33	22.00%
Total	150	100.00%

Table 2.
Number of subjects per COPD stage.

The duration of COPD for patients in this study is shown in **Figure 1**. The average length of the disease is 25.9 years ±11.9. Analysis of the available literature yielded similar data, where the duration of COPD in subjects from group A was 15.6 years, and in subjects from group B 25.5 years [22].

The above statistics show that the development of COPD is generally preceded by a long history of smoking. Typically, nicotine weakens the line of defense in the lungs, the defense systems are activated, mucus secretion increases, and obstruction develops that is initially reversible but eventually becomes irreversible. In addition, airway distortion occurs due to loss of alveolar support and destruction of alveolar septa. For all this, it takes many years for the disease to develop to its full extent, and one of the reasons for development may be insufficient prevention at the primary level of health care.

Quitting smoking can bring many benefits for people with lung diseases. They will be less prone to lung infections and exacerbations of the current condition, they will have fewer hospitalizations, their oxygen levels will be higher and their carbon monoxide levels will return to normal. As many of the symptoms will be alleviated, they will be less likely to be temporarily unable to work [23]. However, according to the results in **Table 3**, the ratio of the number of smokers to ex-smokers among the

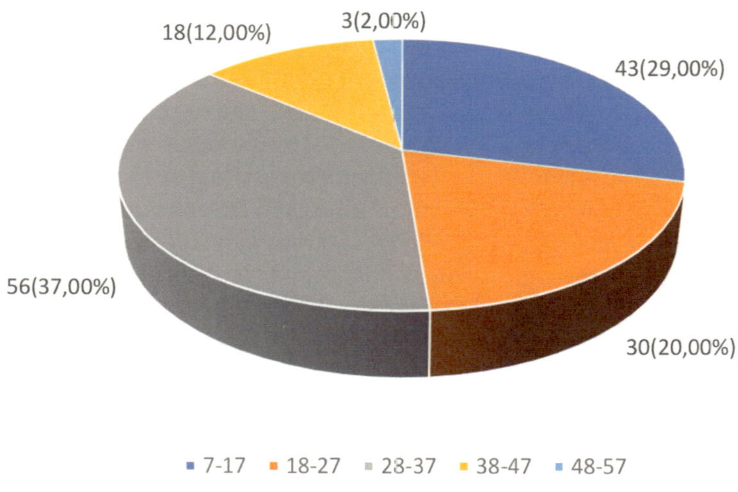

Figure 1.
Duration of COPD in patients (in years).

	Number	Percentage
Smokers	108	72.00%
Ex- smokers	42	28.00%
Total	150	100.00%

Table 3.
Ratio of the number of smokers and ex-smokers among the respondents.

respondents is about 2.6 and, unfortunately, the number of respondents with smoking habits is 108, i.e. 72.00%, with only 42, i.e. 28.00%, ex-smokers.

Results in the available literature are similar to ours [24]. It is very difficult to convince smokers that smoking promotes further reduction of lung function and prevents adequate treatment of any deterioration. Smoking is part of the daily routine for these patients and causes a strong addiction, so smokers are unmotivated to stop smoking. Studies have shown that in COPD and other lung diseases, the most important thing is to stop smoking, not to reduce the number of cigarettes [23].

For people with COPD, neither too little nor too much body mass is desirable because both can lead to worsening of the disease and earlier loss of working ability. Malnutrition is common in COPD patients. Loss of muscle mass and strength of respiratory and skeletal muscles is characteristic of patients with COPD and is an independent predictor that increases the frequency and severity of exacerbations [25].

On the other hand, the loss of muscle mass is often not measurable from the patient's overall weight because it is masked by the accumulation of fat, which can worsen the condition and prognosis.

Table 4 shows that the height distributions of the subjects and the average weight of all patients in each height group. The average height of the male subjects was 176.48 ± 6.90 cm, and that of the female subjects was 163.80 cm ± 9.23 cm. The average weight of the male subjects was 86.52 kg ± 14.98 kg, and the female 73 33 kg ± 11.82 kg. The smallest body mass measured in men was 48 kg, and in

Male/female	Height (cm)	Number of respondents	Avarage weight (kg)
Male	140–150	2	49.50
Male	151–160	13	69.31
Male	161–170	23	73.83
Male	171–180	53	84.94
Male	181–190	14	102.79
Total male		105	82.28
Female	140–150	1	48.00
Female	151–160	3	68.33
Female	161–170	8	68.38
Female	171–180	25	86.64
Female	181–190	8	97.38
Total female		45	83.22

Table 4.
Heights and avarage weight of respondents by gender.

women 49 kg. These results did not differ significantly from those of Šrbič, where the smallest weight was 42 kg in the group with COPD, and the average weight was 74.34 ± 17.70, without gender division [19].

The results of many studies indicate that, in addition to smoking, one of the risk factors for a higher incidence of COPD is exposure to industrial dust and chemicals that are present in workplaces and the working environment. In most cases, these are jobs with special working conditions. In the group of 150 respondents, the type of occupation was: tinsmith, car tinsmith, varnisher, policeman, armorer, pump salesman, manual worker, cook, farmer, bricklayer, storekeeper, hairdresser, cleaner, metal turner, fitter, shoemaker, postman, operator, pedagogue, programmer, social worker, physiotherapist, market seller, security guard, sanitation technician, driver, speech therapist, cashier, architect, and construction worker. These occupations involve workplaces with special working conditions where the respondents are exposed to a wide range of harmful noxious agents. A small number of subjects did not fall into this category, and these are for the most part respondents with a higher professional education who are not exposed to the harmful effects of the group of workers with special working conditions (**Table 5**).

Assessment of working ability through the occupational requirements survey (ORS) is an assessment of the compliance of the health condition of the worker, his physical and mental abilities, with the requirements of jobs and work tasks, as well

Substances	Occupations
Paints	Car varnisher; bricklayer
Dust	Armorer; cleaning lady; NK construction worker; tinsmith; metal turner; baker; assistant cook; carpenter; farmer; storekeeper
Motor oil	Auto tinsmith
Exhaust gases	Auto tinsmith; policeman
Varnishes	Car varnisher; carpenter; bricklayer
Gasoline	Auto tinsmith; farmer; shoemaker
Chemical substances	Cleaning lady; hairdresser; sanitation technician
Weather conditions	Cleaning lady; policeman
Shift work	Civil servants; policeman; nurse
Work at heights	Electrical fitter; construction worker
Lifting loads over 25 kg	Manual worker
Micro climate conditions	Tinsmith; manual worker; fitter; metal turner; market seller; farmer
Glue	Shoemaker
Heat	Baker
Additives	Baker
Evaporation	Sanitation technician
Pesticides	Farmer
Fertilizer	Farmer
Temperature change	Baker; merchant

Table 5.
Workplace conditions in relation to harmful substances and microclimate.

as with the conditions of work and the working environment. Since the physiological and psychophysiological capabilities of the worker and the physiological demands of the workplace are constantly changing, the assessment of working ability is not a static activity but a continuous process that follows the worker and the working conditions at his workplace during his entire working life, starting from the first choice of title, the preliminary examination upon starting work, and regular periodic examinations, all the way to the evaluation of the remaining work capacity. Working ability as a specific activity of occupational medicine is primarily a preventive medical activity with the aim of preserving health and working ability, i.e. preventing the occurrence of disability, reducing the number of occupational diseases and injuries at work, and increasing safety and productivity at work [26].

Certain jobs are associated with greater risk due to the exposure of workers to various chemical, physical, and biological hazards. If a worker with COPD works in jobs where harmful emissions into the working environment occur during the work process, then that worker is at risk of health detriments.

Table 6 shows the number of subjects in our study in each COPD category whose ability to work was or was not compromised by the disease. A total of 73 workers, or 48.67%, had preserved work capacity, and 77 workers, or 51.33%, had reduced work capacity. Preserved working ability is the highest in groups A and B, and decreased in groups C and D. This study was done to compare the working ability of subjects suffering from COPD divided into groups according to the GOLD classification, because no more recent data could be found in the available literature, except for the study of Obiljević et al., which indicate that the evaluation of work ability of respondents with COPD limits work ability [27].

Given that COPD shows a significant increase in morbidity and mortality and that in the next 20 years a further increase in incidence is predicted, the aforementioned will bring about changes in working ability and longer absences from work of patients [28]. Kuhajd's doctoral dissertation "Risk factors affecting the outcome of respiratory rehabilitation in patients with COPD" indicated that in subjects with a disease duration of less than 10 years, rehabilitation results are excellent and amount to 77.3%. The success of the rehabilitation was tested over FEV 1, 6 minute walk test, "CAT" questionnaire and "mMRC" questionnaire [29]. That result is why it is necessary at the level of primary health care to apply prevention measures in a timely manner and determine guidelines in the fight against smoking, as well as risk assessment in workplaces.

Spirometric testing should be done in all people who are long-term smokers and who complain of cough and expectoration because early detection of the disease and the start of treatment improve the quality of life, prevent a decline in lung function and delay the onset of comorbidities [30].

Disease severity	Ability to work preserved	%	Reduced working capacity	%
A	33	22.00%	0	0.00%
B	38	25.33%	2	1.33%
C	2	1.33%	42	28.00%
D	0	0.00%	33	22.00%
Total	73	48.67%	77	51.33%

Table 6.
Change in work ability in patients with COPD.

Disease severity	Number of patients	Percentage of Number of patients	FVC mean value %	FVC mean value L	FEV1 mean value %	FEV1 mean value L
A	33	22.00%	75.06%	2.98	61.32%	1.99
B	40	26.67%	70.08%	2.68	55.41%	1.74
C	44	29.33%	53.55%	2.00	47.49%	1.48
D	33	22.00%	44.50%	1.95	38.82%	1.35
Total	150	100.00%				

Table 7.
Comparison of COPD stages in relation to spirometry.

Table 7 compares the stage of COPD to spirometry (which is the gold standard for diagnosing COPD) results from this study's subjects. The lowest values of FVC and FEV1 were obtained by subjects from stage D according to GOLD, and the mean value of FVC was 44.50% (1.95 L). The mean value of FEV1 was 38.82% (1.35 L). These values are similar to results from other studies. Škrbić reported an FEV1 for COPD patients of 1.43 L [19], while Fernández-Villar reported an average value of 40.30% [31].

Figure 2 showed the analysis of the working ability of COPD patients in relation to gender for our study. The percentage of respondents with reduced work ability was higher in male respondents and amounted to 41.33%, and in women it was 10.00%.

The results fit with the analysis of workplaces where more "male" occupations exposed the respondents to the harmful effects of the workplace.

Figure 3 shows the number of respondents who had reduced and preserved working ability in three age groups, 40–50, 51–60, and 61–70 years old. The age group with the highest percentage of reduced ability (35.33%) was 61–70 years (53 respondents).

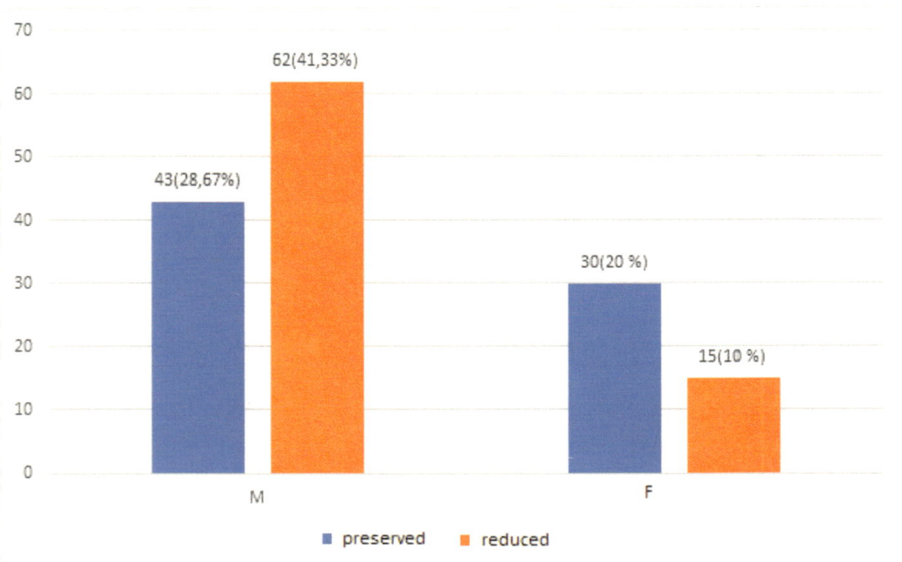

Figure 2.
Changes in working ability of respondents with COPD in relation to gender.

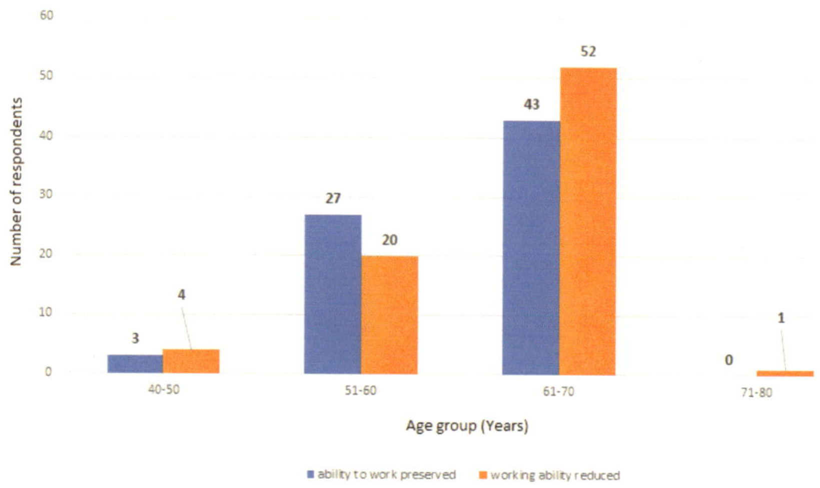

Figure 3.
Change in work ability of respondents with COPD in relation to age.

The average duration of COPD was 31.83 ± 8.79 years for respondents with reduced working capacity and 19.75 ± 10.35 years for respondents with preserved working capacity. A histogram of the number of patients in the preserved and reduced categories in each duration range is shown in **Figure 4**.

Figure 5 shows the number of respondents with reduced and preserved working capacity in each of the four ABCD test categories, None of the respondents in Group A had reduced work capacity. Only 5% of those in Group B had reduced work

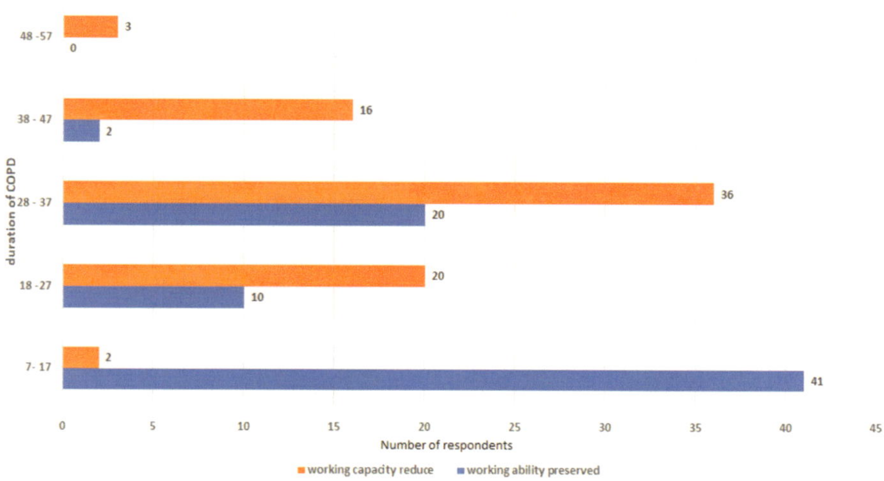

Figure 4.
Change in working capacity in relation to duration of COPD.

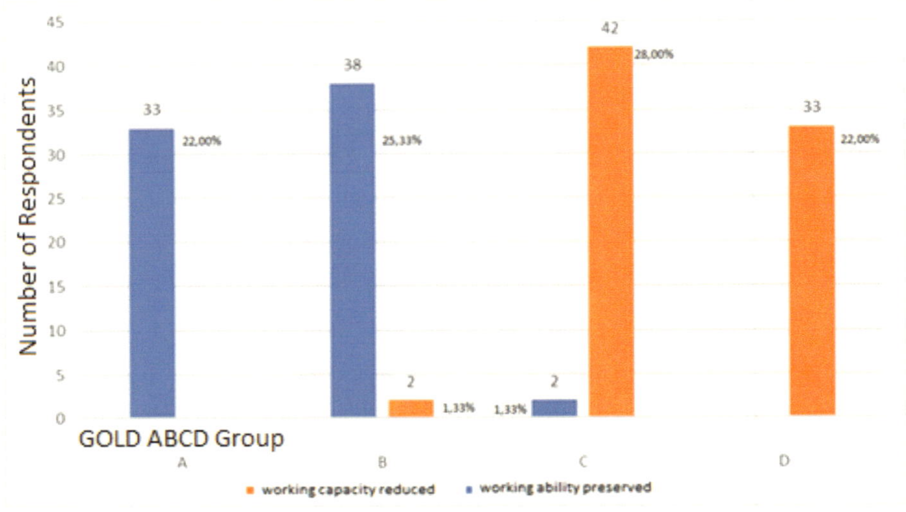

Figure 5.
Altered working capacity in relation to the severity of the disease.

capacity. The vast majority of those in Group C had reduced capacity, and all respondents in Group D had reduced capacity. Overall, work ability was reduced in 77 subjects, i.e. 51.33%, and preserved in 73 subjects. We could not obtain data from other studies on work ability in relation to the duration of COPD and its severity. Groups A and B include subjects who rarely have exacerbations of the disease and who respond best to rehabilitation measures. In stage A, doctors at the primary level of health care play an important role in preventing and preventing exacerbations of the disease and thus reducing the number of lost working days because early detection and recognition of risk factors can be of great importance in preventing the onset of COPD and in preventing the reduction of working capacity.

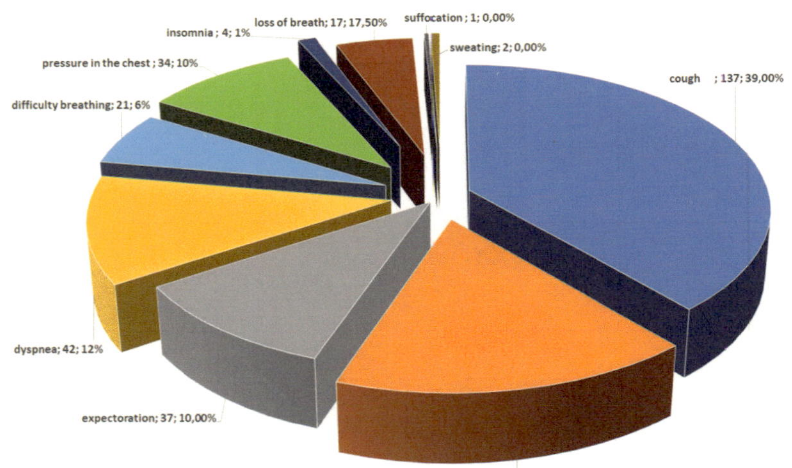

Figure 6.
Distribution of COPD symptoms by frequency.

Figure 6 shows the distribution of COPD symptoms among respondents. Cough occurs in the largest number of respondents n = 137. The next most frequent symptom was fatigue (n = 59), followed by dyspnea (n = 42), expectoration (n = 37) and chest pressure (n = 34). Other symptoms occur in a smaller number of respondents and include difficulty breathing, loss of breath, sweating, insomnia and suffocation.

Of our examinees, 75 had reduced working capacity, and the leading symptom was cough. The same symptom occurred in 52 respondents with preserved work ability. All the leading symptoms occurred in the largest number of respondents with reduced working capacity. As already stated, the largest number of respondents worked in environments with special working conditions and were exposed to workplace hazards that caused increased bronchial secretion and, as a result, prolonged coughing. Symptoms of COPD vary and depend on the stage of the disease. Coughing clears the airways of mucus. Chronic cough is usually the first sign of illness. At first it occurs in the morning occasionally, and later on daily. The cough is generally mild at first and is often mistaken for a "normal" smoker's cough, even though it is not a normal cough. In case of infection, cough is indicated and accompanied by expectoration of yellow or green secretion [31, 32]. Dyspnea is difficulty breathing or shortness of breath. As with cough, dyspnea is accompanied by a limited ability to move due to fatigue, and therefore a limited ability to work during that period. In advanced stages of the disease, dyspnea occurs even at rest. Chest pressure is tightness and a feeling of being unable to breathe.

Table 8 lists the more frequent exacerbations that are associated with absenteeism from work and temporary work incapacity.

Figure 7 showed preserved working capacity within each workplace environment. All such environments were clerical workplaces, where there are no harmful noxious agents and which are not workplaces with increased risk.

Figure 8 shows the number of respondents with reduced working ability in the various workplaces. Reduced capacity respondents were mostly exposed to harmful noxious agents at the workplace.

Figure 9 shows preserved and reduced capacity for smokers and ex-smokers. In the smoker category the numbers of respondents with preserved and reduced working capacity were both 54. In the group of ex-smokers, working ability was reduced in 23 subjects, and preserved in 19.

Absence from work due to illness or injury is considered temporary incapacity for work, during which the employee is entitled to salary compensation. Due to exacerbation of the disease (worsening), 131 respondents were on sick leave for up to 42 days during 1 year, and 73 respondents were absent from work due to illness for more than 42 days. The largest number of absences from work is concentrated in groups C and D, because their exacerbations are more severe and more frequent. This concentration is an indication that COPD significantly affects work ability. Which was the aim of our study. We wanted to draw attention to how important the workplace and work environment are for people diagnosed with COPD. Due to the accompanying manifestations of the disease, people with COPD cannot do heavy physical work, cannot work with chemical irritants, under masks, in a smoky area due to reduced lung volume, cough, ease of fatigue and loss of strength.

People suffering from COPD represent a burden for the Health Insurance Funds due to frequent exacerbations of the disease when therapy and in some cases hospital treatment is required. According to data from the White Book of the European Respiratory Association (ERS White Book) for the year 2011, obstructive diseases (COPD and asthma) had the largest share in total, direct, and indirect costs for

Cough	Fatigue	Expectoration	Dyspnea	Difficulty breathing	Chest pressure	Insomnia	Lose breath	Choking	Weating	Working ability
52	12	8	0	3	20	0	14	0	1	% Preserved
34.67	8.00	5.33	0.00	2.00	13.33	0.00	9.33	0.00	0.67	% Preserved
75	45	30	39	20	14	4	4	1	2	% Reduced
50.00	30.00	20.00	26.00	13.33	9.33%	2.67	2.67	0.67	1.33	% Reduced

Table 8.
Change in working ability in relation to the difficulties of the respondents.

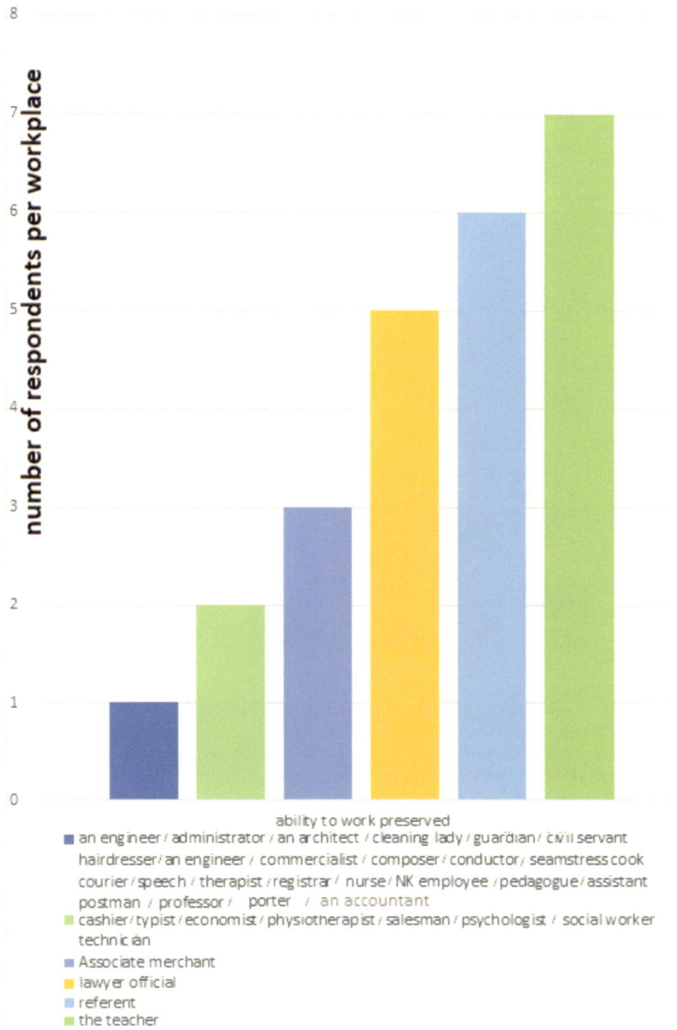

Figure 7.
Ability to work preserved.

respiratory diseases [17]. Total direct costs for respiratory diseases in 2011 amounted to 55 billion euros. Of that amount, COPD is responsible for 23.3 billion euros. In relation to indirect costs amounting to 41.4 billion euros, COPD is responsible for more than half of this amount, i.e. 25.1 billion euros. The cost of treating people with COPD in the United States was $38.6 billion for the same period [33, 34].

COPD represents a major public health problem in the world, and in our country as well, given that it has a high prevalence (up to 600 million patients worldwide), high morbidity (a frequent cause of hospitalization, which accounts for over 75% of the total costs for COPD), high mortality (the fourth leading cause of death), and huge treatment costs (they amount to 2–5 times more than the costs of asthma treatment). Nowadays, there is a significant increase in costs for the treatment of chronic lung diseases in the total costs of health care. The more severe the chronic disease according to GOLD, the higher the direct and indirect costs of treatment. Indirect

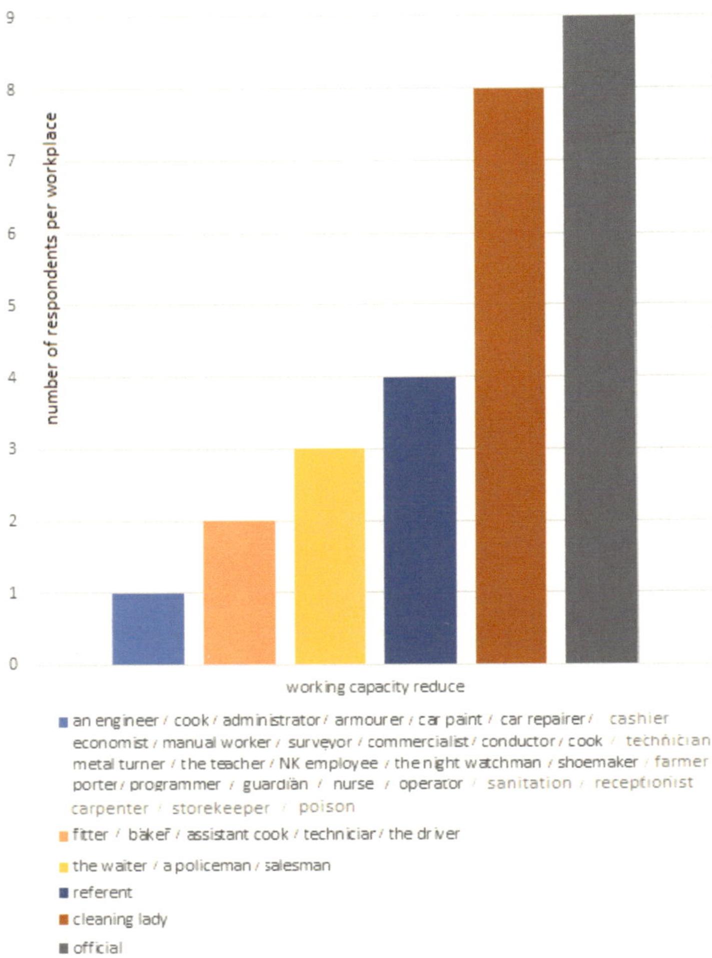

Figure 8.
Working capacity reduce.

costs include loss of ability to work, absence from work, and sick leave, i.e., the period of time for which the employee has the right not to work and to be paid compensation for that time due to inability to work.

Since human capital is often the most important national asset for developing countries, the indirect costs of COPD could be a serious threat to their economies. This group of patients should be the focus of attention of workers, employers and doctors, as well as health and pension insurance funds. In more severe cases, the costs of prevention are many times lower than the costs of treatment, and as such the WHO recommends them for implementation because, from a social perspective, prevention and interventions focused on disease control and slowing the progression of the disease and strengthening work capacity would save costs in COPD, including financial expenses in the category of direct costs-hospitalization and indirect costs.

COPD is also preventable through mitigation of influencing risk factors. In this sense, many strategies are implemented today, such as campaigns against smoking and exposure to tobacco smoke, reduction of air pollution and exposure to harmful substances in the workplace [35].

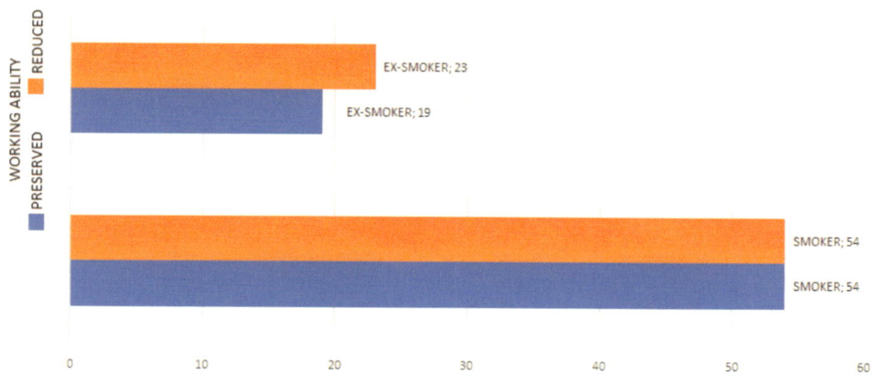

Figure 9.
Working capacity in relation to nicotine abuse.

It is necessary to combine preventive and curative medicine, which reduces the possibility of aggravation and provides an even better overview of the health status of workers, when assessing the work capacity of patients with COPD [12, 36]. Also, ORS should have its role at all levels of prevention (primary, secondary and tertiary) of work-related health disorders [37].

4. Conclusions

This study examined the influence of the work environment and work ability in people diagnosed with chronic obstructive pulmonary disease. The largest number of respondents worked at places with difficult working conditions and were exposed to workplace hazards that caused increased bronchial secretion and, as a result, prolonged coughing. These environments are associated with more frequent exacerbations that are associated with being absent from work - temporary work incapacity and overall loss of workforce capability. The more severe the chronic disease according to GOLD, the higher the direct and indirect costs of treatment.

It is necessary to raise awareness about the primary prevention of all risk factors that lead to exacerbation of COPD because the costs of prevention are many times lower than the costs of treatment in more severe cases and as such WHO recommends them for implementation [14, 15, 17].

Conflict of interest

The authors declare no conflict of interest.

Author details

Jasmina Biscevic-Tokic[1*], Zurifa Ajanovic[2], Sanja Brekalo-Lazarevic[3] and Nedim Tokic[4]

1 Medical Faculty of Sarajevo, Department of Occupational Health, Institute of Occupational Medicine of Canton Sarajevo, Sarajevo, Bosnia and Herzegovina

2 Medical Faculty of Sarajevo, Department of Human Anatomy, Bosnia and Herzegovina

3 Medical Faculty of Sarajevo, Department of Occupational Health, Bosnia and Herzegovina

4 Emergency Medicine Clinic, University Clinical Center in Sarajevo, Bosnia and Herzegovina

*Address all correspondence to: jasmina.biscevic@mf.unsa.ba

References

[1] Global Initiative for Chronic Obstructive Lung Disease: The Changes Made. Cureus. 24 Jun 2019;**11**(6):e4985. DOI: 10.7759/cureus.4985

[2] Vogelmeier CF, Criner GJ, Martinez FJ, Anzueto A, Barnes PJ, Bourbeau J, et al. Global strategy for the diagnosis, management, and prevention of chronic obstructive lung disease 2017 report. Respirology. 2017;**22**:575-601

[3] Nakawah MO, Hawkins C, Barbandi F. Asthma, chronic obstructive pulmonary disease (COPD), and the overlap syndrome. Journal of the American Board of Family Medicine. 2013;**26**(4):470-477

[4] Rabe KF, Hurd S, Anzueto A, i sur. Global strategy for the diagnosis, management, and prevention of chronic obstructive pulmonary disease: GOLD executive summary. American Journal of Respiratory and Critical Care Medicine. 2007;**176**:532-555

[5] Macan J, Zavalić M. Ocjena Radne Sposobnosti u Medicini Rada. Zagreb: Medicinska naklada; 2019

[6] Žuškin Š i. Medicina Rada i Okoliša. Zagreb: Medicinska Naklada; 2002

[7] Mustajbegović J, Milošević M, Brborović H. Medicina Rada i Sporta. Zagreb: Medicinska Naklada; 2018

[8] Stallberg B, Janson C, Johansson G, et al. Management, morbidity and mortality of COPD during an 11-year period: An observational retrospective epidemiological register study in Sweden (PATHOS). Primary Care Respiratory Journal. 2014;**23**(1):38-45

[9] Aranđelović M, Jovanović J. Medicina Rada. Niš: Medicinski fakultet; 2009

[10] Wacker ME, Jorres RA, Schulz H, Heinrich J, Karrasch S, Karch A, et al. Direct and indirect costs of COPD and its comorbidities: Results from the German COSYCONET study. Respiratory Medicine. 2016;**111**:39-46

[11] Dal Negro RW. COPD: The annual cost-of-illness during the last two decades in Italy, and its mortality predictivity power. Healthcare (Basel). 2019;**7**(1):35

[12] Patel AR, Patel AR, Singh S, Singh S, Khawaja I. Global initiative for chronic obstructive lung disease. Cureus. 24 Jun 2019;**11**(6):e4985. DOI: 10.7759/cureus.4985

[13] Kirsch F, Schramm A, Schwarzkopf L, Lutter JI, Szentes B, Huber M, et al. Direct and indirect costs of COPD progression and its comorbidities in a structured disease management program: Results from the LQ-DMP study. Respiratory Research. 10 Oct 2019

[14] Huber MB, Wacker ME, Vogelmeier CF, Leidl R. Excess costs of comorbidities in chronic obstructive pulmonary disease: A systematic review. PLoS One. 2015

[15] Chen W, FitzGerald JM, Sin DD, Sadatsafavi M. Excess economic burden of comorbidities in COPD: A 15-year population-based study. The European Respiratory Journal. 2017;**50**:1700393. DOI: 10.1183/13993003.00393-2017

[16] Jansson SA, Backman H, Stenling A, Lindberg A, Ronmark E, Lundback B. Health economic costs of COPD in Sweden by disease severity—has it changed during a ten years period. Respiratory Medicine. 2013;**107**:1931-1938

[17] European Respiratory Society (ERS). European Lung White Book – Chapter 2:

The Economic Burden of Lung Disease. 2016;**2**:26 [Accessed: October 12, 2016]

[18] Ljubičić Đ. Sveučilište u zagrebu medicinski fakultet [Internet]. [cited 2023 Nov 13]. Available from: https://core.ac.uk/download/pdf/185265755.pdf

[19] Škrbić D. Metabolički sindrom kod pacijenata sa hroničnom opstruktivnom bolesti pluća i bronhiektazijama. Novi Sad; 2015. Available from: https://hdl.handle.net/21.15107/rcub_nardus_4716

[20] Maričić L. Procjena endotelne disfunkcije kod oboljelih od kronične opstruktivne plućne bolesti. Zagreb: Godine; 2015

[21] Rizvic E. Svjetski dan kronične opstruktivne plucne bolesti (KOPB) [Internet]. ZZJZ FBiH. 2016 [cited 2023 Nov 13]. Available from: https://www.zzjzfbih.ba/svjetski-dan-kronicne-opstruktivne-plucne-bolesti-kopb/

[22] Pavličević I, Perić I, Glavaški M. Ispitivanje komorbiditeta u bolesnika s kroničnom opstrukcijskom plućnom bolesti. Hrvatska: Medicinski fakultet Sveučilišta u Splitu, Klinički bolnički centar Split;

[23] Pušenje za vrijeme plućne bolesti Zašto bih trebao/la prestati pušiti? Trenutne prednosti Dugoročne prednosti [Internet]. [cited 2023 Nov 13]. Available from: https://europeanlung.org/wp-content/uploads/2021/01/smoking-when-you-have-a-croatian.pdf

[24] Faktori rizika koji utiču na ishod respiratorne rehabilitacije kod pacijenata sa hroničnom opstruktivnom bolesti pluća doktorska disertacija [Internet]. [cited 2023 Nov 13]. Available from: https://nardus.mpn.gov.rs/bitstream/handle/123456789/6840/Disertacija146787770176168.pdf

[25] Gazdek D, Samardžić S. Croatian smoke-free law and smoking habits among employees of health care facilities in Koprivnica-Križevci County. Croatian Medical Journal. Aug 2013;**54**(4):407-410

[26] Bojana Knežević. Ocjena Radne Sposobnosti u Medicini Rada. Available from: http://zastitanaradu.dashofer.hr/33/18.7.2016

[27] Okiljević Z, Jovančević Drvenica M, Kopitović I, Kovačević T, Trivić B. The algorithm for the assessment of functional work capacity of railway workers with chronic obstructive pulmonary disease COPD. Praxis Medica. 2014;**43**(2):55-59

[28] Rabe KF, Hurd S, Anzueto A, i sur. Global strategy for the diagnosis, management, and prevention of chronic obstructive pulmonary disease: GOLD executive summary. American Journal of Respiratory and Critical Care Medicine. 2007;**176**:532-555

[29] Kuhajda D. Faktori Rizika Koji utiču na ishod Respiratorne Rehabilitacije kod Pacijenata sa Hroničnom Opstruktivnom Bolesti Pluća. Novi Sad: Doktorska Disertacija; 2016

[30] Agusti A, Hogg JC. Update on the pathogenesis of chronic obstructive pulmonary disease. The New England Journal of Medicine. 26 Sep 2019;**381**(13):1248-1256

[31] Fernández-Villar A, Represas-Represas C, Mouronte-Roibás C, Ramos-Hernández C, Sara F-GA, López-Campos J. Reliability and usefulness of spirometry performed during admission for COPD exacerbation. PLoS One. 2018;**13**(3):e0194983

[32] Fisk M et al. Clinical characteristics and management of patients with an inaccurate diagnosis of chronic obstructive

pulmonary disease (copd) in primary care; results from the welsh national copd primary care audit. Thorax. 2017

[33] Vos T, Flaxman AD, Naghavi M, i sur. Years lived with disability (YLDs) for 1160 sequelae of 289 diseases and injuries 1990-2010: A systematic analysis for the global burden of disease study 2010. Lancet. 2012;**380**:2163-2196

[34] Lopez-Campos JL, Tan W, Soriano JB. Global burden of COPD. Respirology. 2016;**21**:14-23

[35] Čekerevac I. Sistemski efekti hronične opstruktivne bolesti pluća [PhD Thesis]. Medicinski Fakultet: Univerzitet u Kragujevcu; 2009,616.24-036.1:616-008

[36] Osmanagic A. Hronična opstruktivna plućna bolest. Kontinuirana Medicinska Edukacija

[37] Agarwal AK, Raja A, Brown BD. Chronic Obstructive Pulmonary Disease (COPD). 2020

Chapter 6

Balance Impairments in COPD

Qurat Ul Ain, Yasha Sajjad and Tahzeem Riaz

Abstract

Chronic Obstructive Pulmonary disease (COPD) not only impacts pulmonary function but has deleterious impacts on musculoskeletal system and balance of patients. In any individual, balance is the result of interplay between musculoskeletal, neurological, and environmental aspects, and disturbance in any one or more can affect overall balance control. In COPD, balance impairments have been increasingly reported over the past few years. There are many multifactorial dimensions behind this rising trajectory. Berg balance scale, time up and go, single leg stance, and mini-balance evaluation system have been established as reasonable, valid, and effective tools for screening balance impairments in COPD. Additionally, amalgamation of balance training, tai chi exercises, and breathing exercises in a pulmonary rehabilitation regime have proven to be effective in improving balance and reducing fall risks in patients living with COPD.

Keywords: COPD, balance, balance impairments, pulmonary, physical therapy

1. Introduction

Chronic Obstructive Pulmonary Disease (COPD) is a chronic respiratory ailment characterized by its progressive nature, which entails a gradual deterioration of lung function, leading to airflow restriction and respiratory distress. Globally, COPD looms as a substantial public health challenge, ranking as the fourth leading cause of mortality in developed nations, and projections suggest it may ascend to the third position by 2030 [1]. This debilitating condition exhibits symptoms of bronchitis, emphysema, and asthma (**Figure 1**), and it exacts a formidable toll on individuals grappling with it, manifesting through a spectrum of distressing symptoms (**Table 1**). The most prevalent among these are a persistent and often productive cough, episodes of breathlessness that can be triggered by even minimal exertion, and the production of thick, viscous sputum. Additionally, although less frequent, symptoms like a constricting sensation in the chest, feelings of chest congestion, and audible wheezing can significantly impact one's quality of life.

Beyond its systemic manifestations, COPD exerts a profound impact on the holistic well-being of affected individuals. This malady precipitates a notable decline in exercise tolerance, making routine activities increasingly challenging. Peripheral muscles progressively weaken, diminishing overall physical performance and functional mobility. Moreover, recent scientific investigations have unveiled an intriguing facet of COPD - a notable impairment in balance control, which can further exacerbate the difficulties faced by those living with this condition [1–6].

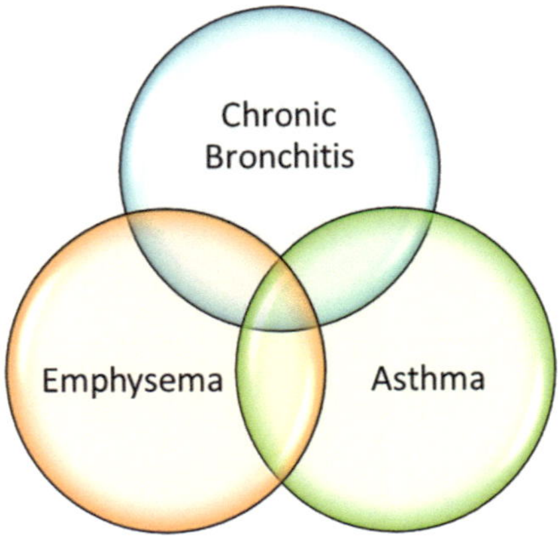

Figure 1.
COPD as an amalgamation of three pathologies.

Decreased exercise tolerance
Progressive peripheral muscular weakness
Diminution of functional mobility
Activities of daily living in jeopardy
Balance impairments

Table 1.
Physical manifestations of COPD.

2. The science of balance control

According to Kisner et al., "Balance is a complex motor control task involving the detection and integration of sensory information to assess the position and motion of the body in space and the execution of appropriate musculoskeletal responses to control body position within the context of the environment and task. Thus, balance control requires the interplay of the nervous and musculoskeletal systems and contextual effects" (**Figure 2**) [7].

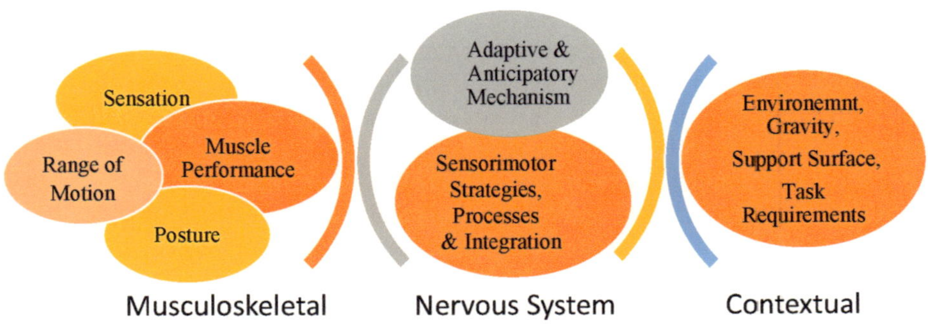

Figure 2.
Integration of three systems for maintaining balance.

3. Balance assessment in COPD

Several tests are available to screen for balance impairments within populations. The most common of these are time up and go (TUG), single leg stance, Berg Balance Scale (BBS), and mini and full balance evaluation systems. To assess the likelihood of a fall, it is recommended to use shorter balance assessment tests, so that fall does not occur during assessment. Whenever a health care provider comes across an older adult, they need to ask some specific questions that have been identified in several clinical practice guidelines (**Figure 3**). These questions include:

1. Have you experienced fall in last 1 year?

2. Do feel unsteady while getting up, standing or walking?

If the answer to these questions is yes, then the balance screening and evaluation tests should be used.

3.1 Berg balance scale test

The BBS test is widely used and can be administered by a physical therapist in a time span of almost 15 minutes. It has a cumulative score of 56, and values less than 45 indicate increased risk of fall. It measures a vast variety of performance based tasks ranging from getting up from a chair to standing on one leg. The healthcare provider will guide you through a set of tasks, grading your performance on a scale from 0 to 4 for each. The cumulative scores result from evaluating your ability to complete 14 specific movements:

1. Transition from sitting to standing.

2. Stand without support.

3. Sit without support.

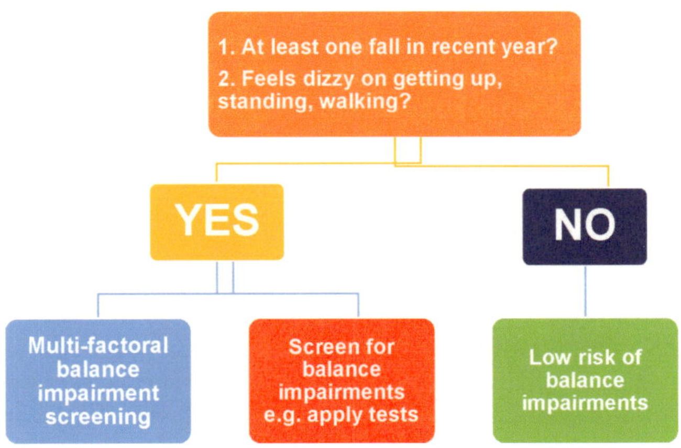

Figure 3.
Summary of balance screening protocol extracted from different CPGs reported in a research conducted by Beauchamp et al. [8].

4. Move from standing to sitting.

5. Transfer between chairs.

6. Stand with closed eyes.

7. Maintain a standing position with feet together.

8. Reach forward with an outstretched arm.

9. Retrieve an object from the floor.

10. Turn and glance behind you.

11. Rotate in a full circle.

12. Place each foot alternately on a stool in front of you.

13. Stand without support with one foot directly in front of the other.

14. Balance on one leg for as long as possible [9].

However, it considers neither cognitive functionality and its influence on balance nor the impact of unanticipated perturbations on balance. Those two factors are included in the mini-balance evaluations systems (mini-BES) test, which is also used in clinical practices to conduct a balance assessment in COPD patients. Balance assessment while maintaining cognitive functionality is checked in mini-BES test through walking with pivot turns, stepping over obstacles and utilizing time up and go with dual-tasking e.g. ask the subject to count from any number and then say go, or ask the subject to count backwards from 100 to 90 or between any two numbers. Note the speed while performing these activities. Conversely, unanticipated perturbations' impact is checked in the form of compensatory stepping strategy that will be adapted after removal of backward, lateral and forward external support. Patients with moderate balance disorders tend to take several steps instead of one big step and, in severe balance issues take no step at all and fall spontaneously. The maximum score of the mini-BES test is 28 [10]. After comprehensive analysis of psychometric properties, both the BBS and mini-BES test are recommended to assess patients with COPD.

3.2 Time up and go test

The short duration of the TUG test makes it preferable for COPD patients when functional disability is a concern. The subject is asked to stand from a seated position, walk to a marker 3 meters away, return to the seat, and sit back down (**Figure 4**). The time required for this activity is the TUG value. Albarrati et al. recommend a value of 8.42 seconds to indicate normal functional activity, while they found an average TUG value of 12 seconds in their older adult COPD patients and found a significant difference between COPD patients and non-COPD subjects in the four age groups that they studied (<49, 50–59, 60–69, and > 79 years of age) [11].

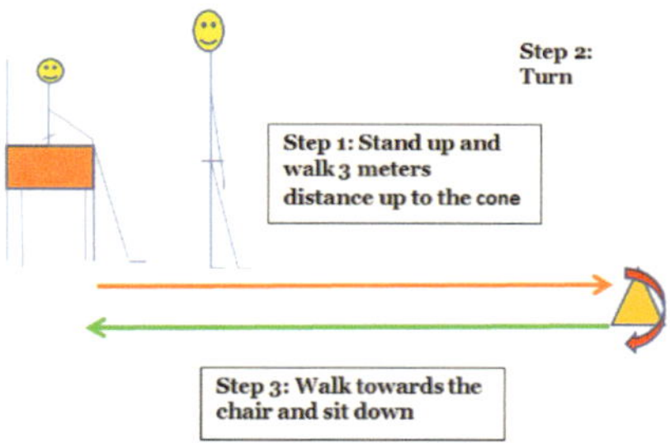

Figure 4.
Time up & go test for measuring time taken to walk back and forth over 3 meters distance. A time > 13 seconds taken to complete this test indicates risk of fall.

Values for TUG and frailty index were greater in COPD patients with frequent exacerbations of symptoms. In addition, a retrospective study showed that TUG has excellent reliability and accuracy for determining the risk of fall in patients with COPD [12, 13].

3.3 Single leg stance

The *Single Leg Stance (SLS)* test has been shown to be most promising clinical assessment tool in patients with COPD. This test provides results as accurate as those given by long balance-related screening tests. But in a clinical setting where time is short and efficiency is given priority, this test is more acceptable than other tests [14]. The single-leg stance involves standing on one leg without assistance, with eyes open and arms placed on the hips. Timing begins when one foot is lifted from the floor and ends when it touches either the ground or the standing leg, or when an arm leaves the hips. Individuals unable to maintain this stance for a minimum of 5 seconds face an elevated risk of experiencing injurious falls [15].

3.4 Modified Romberg test and Romberg test

The Romberg test includes standing on firm surface without shoes and with feet together. This activity is timed, first with eyes open, and then with closed eyes. Minimum limit is 30 seconds to hold the position if balance issues are absent [16]. The modified Romberg test assesses an individual's capacity to stand without assistance through four distinct test conditions. These conditions are specifically crafted to evaluate the sensory inputs essential for maintaining balance, including the vestibular system, vision, and proprioception. This test examines participants with both open and closed eyes on firm and compliant surfaces. When eyes are open on a firm surface, visual, proprioceptive, and vestibular systems are assessed. Closing the eyes on the firm surface focuses on vestibular and proprioceptive systems. On the foam pad with open eyes, visual and vestibular systems are challenged, while closing the eyes on the foam pad specifically targets the vestibular system. Presently, the definition of test failure involves a subject being required to open their eyes, moving their arms or feet to regain stability, or starting to fall and necessitating operator intervention to sustain balance within a 30-second timeframe. This test is marked as pass if all four conditions have successfully completed by participant, and marked fail if any one condition has been failed [17].

Test name	Purpose	Time Taken
Berg Balance Scale (BBS)	Core balance	15 minutes
Mini-Balance evaluation system (BES) Test	Core balance	15 minutes
Time up & go	Fall risk	<5 minutes
Single Leg Stance (SLS)	Fall risk	<5 minutes

Table 2.
Characteristics and validity of balance screening tests in COPD patients [8].

3.5 Fall efficacy scale-international (FES-I)

The FES-I comprises 16 questions designed to evaluate participants' apprehension regarding falling while engaging in 16 distinct ADLs (cleaning, bathing, shopping, cooking, dressing, getting up or out of chair, cooking, using stairs, walking in neighborhood, reaching overhead or to the ground, picking up the phone before it stops ringing, walking on wet grounds, paying a visit to friend or relative, walking in crowded regions, walking on uneven surfaces, slopes, and attending a social gathering). Each item on the FES-I is graded on a 4-point scale (1 = not at all concerned to 4 = very concerned). The cumulative score spans from 16 to 64, with 16 representing "no concern" and 64 signifying an "extreme concern about falling" while carrying out the activities outlined in the questionnaire [18].

3.6 Six minute walk test

The 6-minute walk test (6MWT) evaluates the distance walked within a 6-minute duration, serving as a sub-maximal assessment of aerobic capacity/endurance [19]. Additionally, if the covered distance is below 331 meters, it signals an increased risk of falls [20].

3.7 Activity specific balance confidence scale

The Activities-specific Balance Confidence (ABC) scale is a structured survey designed to gauge an individual's confidence in ambulatory activities, ensuring they can perform these activities without fear of falling or feeling unsteady. Developed in 1995 by Powell and Myers, the scale comprises 16 questions that assess the individual's confidence levels during various activities. It scores from 0 to 100, 100 indicates maximum confidence for performing ADLs [21].

The characteristics of the commonly used tests are summarized in **Table 2**. All tests have good construct validity in COPD and show statistical significance between high and low risk of fall.

4. The shaky ground: a closer look at balance impairments

When integration of all these systems is disrupted by some underlying pathology, balance problems emerge. However, with aging even normal adults begin to face balance-related issues due to changes in the musculoskeletal system, the nervous system, and the ability to track contextual factors [22].

A study performed by Zahra et al. that included 2004 older individuals without COPD above 60 years from Pakistan showed that 89.67% (1797) failed the modified Romberg Balance Test and 10.33% (207) passed it. Failed candidates are those in which some kind of balance impairment is present. Participants those who failed in phase 2 did not get tested for phase 3 and phase 4, similarly those who fail in phase 3 were not considered for phase 4. 654 out of 2004 failed second phase (32%), 464 out of 1350 failed third phase (34%), and 678 out of 884 people failed in phase 4 (77%). Chi-square test showed p value less than 0.05, showing increasing age was significantly correlated with balance disturbances [23]. In contrast to that, a study by Khan et al. in 2021 conducted on younger women between 18 and 30 years of age showed 98 percent of them passed Romberg test, and only 1.3% failed [24]. Hence, age does play a role in disturbing balances.

Deficiencies in the motor aspects of balance control can be attributed to problems in the musculoskeletal system, such as poor posture, limited joint movement, and weakened muscles, and in the neuromuscular system, such as poor motor coordination and pain. One COPD-related musculoskeletal issue that affects balance is the typical thoracic kyphosis, which shifts the body's center of mass away from the subject's base of support, increasing the risk of losing balance.

In cases where the legs function as closed chains (i.e., with the foot position fixed), limitations in range of motion or muscle strength at one joint can influence the overall posture and balance of the entire limb. For instance, if ankle motion is restricted due to contractures or ankle dorsiflexor weakness, the use of an ankle-based balance strategy is diminished, and the hip and trunk muscles are relied on more strongly for balance control.

In individuals with neurological conditions like stroke, traumatic brain injury, or Parkinson's disease, difficulties in generating sufficient muscle force due to abnormal muscle tone or impaired coordination of motor strategies may restrict their ability to engage the necessary muscles for maintaining balance. Moreover, persistent pain can alter movements, reduce a person's normal stability, and, over time, lead to additional issues with strength and mobility. Addressing these factors is crucial when focusing on rehabilitation for balance and mobility [7]. In COPD, loss of muscular strength and poor posture are believed to be the primary causes for balance impairments.

5. COPD's sneaky move: the unseen tango with balance impairments

People diagnosed with COPD face a notable risk of experiencing falls due to a combination of various factors (**Figure 5**). Among these factors are issues such as poor postural control, weakness in the lower limb muscles, and compromised functional performance. Additionally, individuals with COPD who are able to walk but require a constant oxygen supply may encounter the risk of stumbling over the oxygen lines and experiencing a fall. Research findings have underscored the significance of this concern, indicating that COPD ranks as the second highest chronic pathology associated with falls, trailing only behind osteoarthritis [25]. The incidence rate of falls among individuals with COPD ranges from 25 to 46% [25, 26].

Apart from factors like age, depression, malnutrition, and cognitive problems, faulty postural balance emerges as a major intrinsic risk factor for falls within the COPD population. Understanding the mechanisms behind these balance disorders reveals a complex interplay between sensory input and motor function. When individuals with COPD face postural challenges that disrupt their balance, their trunk

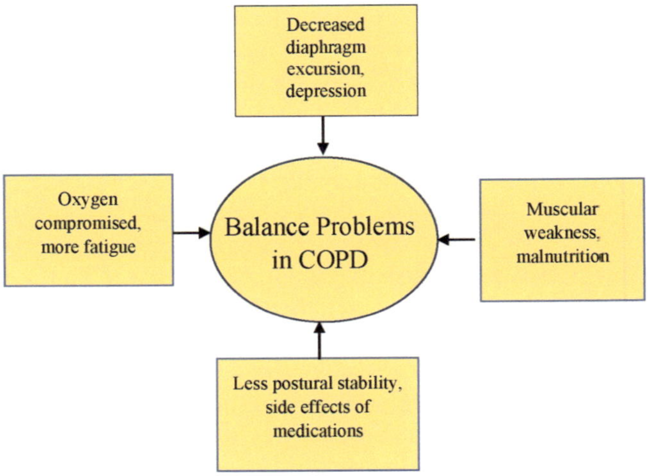

Figure 5.
COPD and its direct impact on balance.

and respiratory muscles, especially the diaphragm, play a crucial role in stabilizing their bodies. However, it is reasonable to suggest that the increased workload on respiratory muscles in COPD may compromise their ability to maintain stable postures.

Moreover, recent research has highlighted specific balance issues in the COPD population, particularly when they engage in more dynamic activities that demand the use of their lower limb muscles. Numerous studies have linked balance difficulties in stable COPD cases to muscular weakness. As the severity of the disease progresses, individuals with COPD experience muscle mass loss, primarily in their thigh muscles. Consequently, these patients endure reduced endurance levels, heightened fatigue, and breathlessness even during minimal exertion. These symptoms limit their daily activities and exercise tolerance, setting in motion a cycle of decreased mobility and functionality.

Lower limb muscular weakness emerges as a non-pulmonary risk factor for falls, yet individuals with COPD face a greater risk of falling compared to the general population. Poor postural control is not exclusive to COPD but is a common concern among the elderly. About 30% of individuals over the age of 60 experiences at least one fall annually, with the incidence rising to 45% among those over 70 [25]. Faulty postural control becomes more pronounced when underlying chronic conditions are present, and COPD is more prevalent in older populations.

Evidence supports the connection between age and faulty postural control in individuals with COPD, which in turn elevates their risk of falls. Other well-established risk factors for falls, including lower limb muscle weakness, labyrinthine disorders, functional dependence, and the inability to regain balance after a stumble, are frequently encountered by COPD patients. While the risk of falls may seem less urgent when compared to the respiratory challenges of COPD, these falls are associated with increased mortality, dependency, reduced physical function, and a diminished quality of life, affecting both COPD patients and the general population. Furthermore, the consequences of falls are economically burdensome for the healthcare system, as they lead to higher mortality and morbidity rates and to functional decline and earlier admission to care facilities. Therefore, reducing the incidence of falls is a crucial goal within the healthcare system [25, 27–35].

Balance issues are not an isolated aspect of the COPD patient's health. They are part of a type of positive feedback system that can lead to acceleration of the decline of a patient's

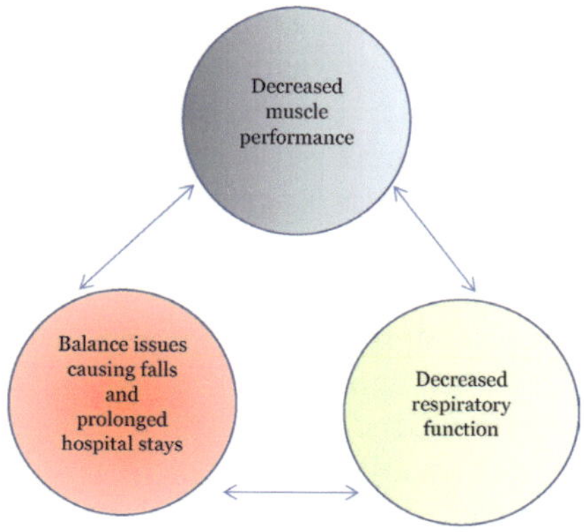

Figure 6.
Vicious cycle of muscle impairments, increased hospital stays, falls and decreased respiratory functions in COPD.

health (**Figure 6**). If a balance issue leads to a fall, it can lead to a hospital stay or otherwise to reduced activity that leads to decreased muscle performance. Decreased muscle performance can then increase the probability of a consecutive fall and reduce respiratory performance. Reduced respiratory performance can further reduce activity, leading to a further decrease in muscle performance and further exacerbating the balance issues.

6. Stepping carefully: COPD's impact on balance unveiled in the research literature

Chuatrakoon et al. [36] conducted a systematic review aimed at identifying balance deficits and evaluating the impact of physiotherapy interventions on patients diagnosed with COPD. This comprehensive review incorporated data from fifteen cross-sectional studies and four Randomized Controlled Trials (RCTs), which were sourced from a variety of reputable electronic databases, including the Cochrane Library, Scopus, PubMed, and CINAHIL. To assess the quality of the included studies, the National Institute of Health (NIH) quality assessment tool was utilized. This assessment indicated that ten of the cross-sectional studies exhibited a moderate to high level of quality, as they achieved an NIH score greater than 7. Additionally, the quality of the RCTs was appraised using the Pedro scale, which indicated that these trials ranged from good to excellent in quality, with Pedro scores ranging from 6 to 9. The key findings of this systematic review underscore the significant presence of balance impairment among individuals suffering from COPD, as determined through various balance assessment tests when compared to the general population. Consequently, the review strongly advocates for the incorporation of balance training as an integral component of physiotherapy rehabilitation programs designed for individuals with COPD, aiming to address and ameliorate their balance issues.

A 2016 study conducted by de Castro et al. [37] examined the differences in functional and static balance between individuals with COPD and a control group without COPD. The study also explored how gender and the severity of COPD might influence balance. The study's findings indicated that COPD patients exhibited poorer static and dynamic balance compared to their healthy counterparts. Notably, gender appeared to play a role, with men performing better in functional balance assessments, while women demonstrated superior results in static balance tests.

Oliveira et al. [38] investigated the extent of fear of falling (FOF) in individuals afflicted with COPD. Additionally, they sought to unravel the intricate nexus between FOF and various factors: the muscular strength exerted during physical activities, the ability to maintain balance, and the maximum level of physical exertion sustainable by COPD patients during any given task. To gauge the participants' FOF, the researchers employed the Falls Efficacy Scale International (FES-I). Meanwhile, the assessment of physical functionality in both the COPD and control groups entailed the use of quadriceps hand-held dynamometry, the Six-minute Walk Test, and the BBS. The findings of their investigation shed light on significant disparities. They observed that, as the severity of COPD increased, individuals exhibited poorer control over their balance and a decline in their ability to carry out everyday activities. This result was corroborated by statistical significance, with a p-value of 0.01. Moreover, those with COPD displayed higher scores on the FES-I, signifying an elevated level of fear of falling ($p < 0.01$) when compared to their healthy counterparts.

Riaz [39] compared balance impairments among COPD and healthy population. They conducted research on 16 patients with diagnosed COPD and 16 healthy adults between ages of 40 to 65 years. An ABC questionnaire was used to gauge the participants' balance confidence while doing complex and daily living tasks. In addition, BBS and TUG were used to assess static and dynamic balance and risk of falls, respectively. Moreover, the impacts of age, gender, and BMI on balance were studied.

BBS scores (< 45 indicates risk of fall) were 33–51 for COPD and 49–56 for healthy people. ABC scores (total 100%) were 63–74.3% for COPD and 66–90.14% for healthy. TUG scores (≤13 sec is normal) were 12–16 seconds for COPD and 7–13 seconds for healthy [36–38].

Comparisons for the BBS ($p < 0.05$), ABC ($p < 0.05$) and TUG ($p < 0.05$) scores between the COPD and healthy subjects were statistically significant, as determined

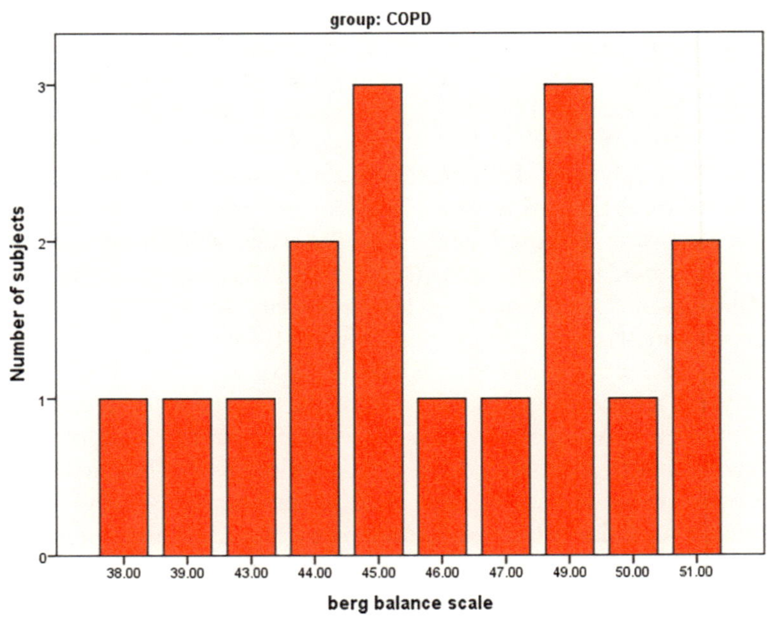

Figure 7.
Bar chart showing berg balance scale scores in COPD (scores: 38–51) (un-reported and additional data from study conducted by Riaz et al.)

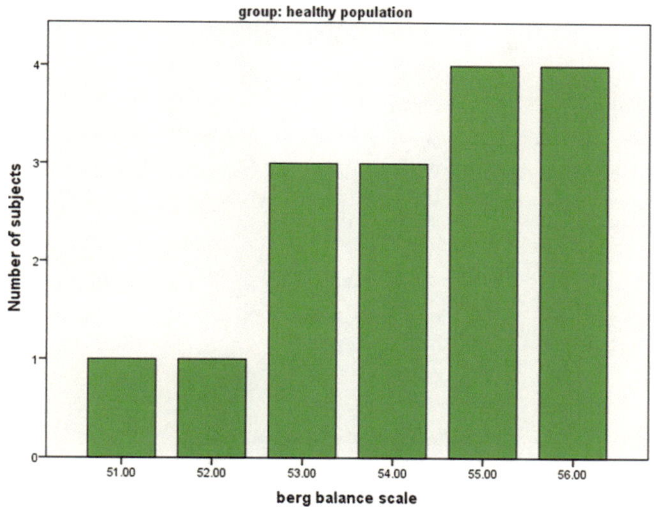

Figure 8.
Bar chart showing berg balance scale scores in healthy population (scores 51–56). (un-reported and additional data from study conducted by Riaz et al.)

from an independent t test. Age and cigarette smoking did not significantly impact the BBS and TUG scores, whereas BMI correlated with all three measures [39].

Additional data provided by Riaz et al. show that BBS was significantly correlated with age (p = 0.02) and smoking (0.03) in the COPD group, and no significant correlation was found between BBS and BMI in COPD patients (p = 0.9). In contrast, BBS in the healthy population was significantly correlated with BMI only, with $p < 0.05$, and no correlation was found with smoking and age, with p = 0.20 & p = 0.24 respectively.

A BBS score greater than 45 indicates the ability to perform functional activities independently without having the risk of fall. None of the COPD patients' scores exceeded 51, and the peak number of participants was recorded at scores of 45 and 49 (**Figure 7**). However, in healthy population BBS score peaks were 55 and 56 (**Figure 8**). Thus, the ability to perform functional activities without experiencing falls is greater for healthy subjects than for COPD patients.

7. Treatment options for balance impairments in COPD

Balance training consists of four main exercises (**Figure 9**). These exercises need to be added to a pulmonary rehabilitation program for COPD, and breathing exercises need to be incorporated in all sessions. Balance training needs to be followed 5 days a week over at least 6–8 weeks to significantly improve the balance of patients with COPD. Tandem walking is placing one foot directly in front of the other in a straight line, aiming to have the heel of the front foot touch the toes of the back foot. If bringing one foot against the other is challenging, strive to get them as close together as possible. Repeat this process four times, covering the 10-foot distance [40]. Then progress by asking the patient to count backwards from 100 to 90 while doing tandem walking. In addition to that, standing is timed on unsteady surfaces such as on foam pads or on wobble boards. It can progress further by removing forward, backward and lateral supports in order to improve reactive balance controls. As far as transition exercises

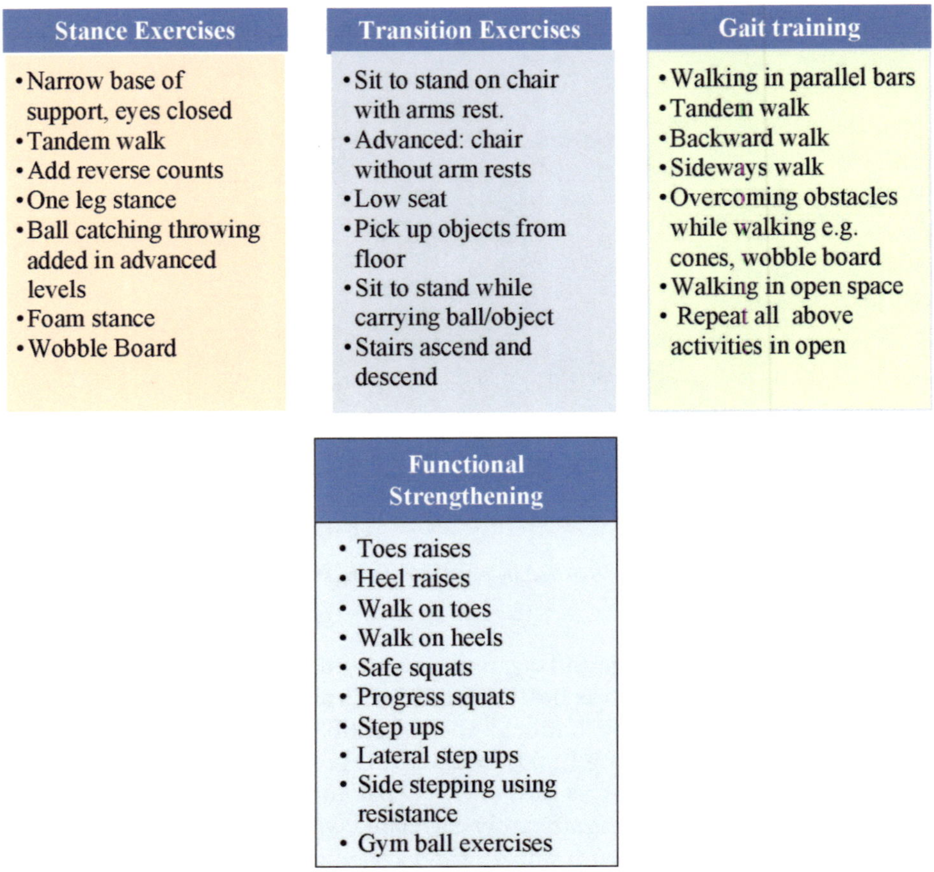

Figure 9.
Balance training program.

are concerned, start by doing sit to stands on chair with arm rests, and it can become more challenging by decreasing height of chair or using a chair without arm rests. Furthermore, functional training can include safe squats, where a chair is used for balance support, the knees are bent up to only 90 degrees, and the patient is advised to go down with the help of the hip instead of putting stress on knees. The squats can progress in intensity by adding a weight to the thighs or hands while performing squats. For a greater challenge, a gym ball can be used in place of a stable chair during the squats.

Beauchamp et al. conducted a randomized controlled trial to examine how a balance-training program influences balance and physical function measures in COPD patients participating in pulmonary rehabilitation (PR). Participants were allocated randomly to either an intervention or control group. The intervention group engaged in balance training three times a week for a duration of 6 weeks, concurrently with PR. The control group exclusively participated in the 6-week PR program. Clinical assessments of balance included the BBS, the BESTest, and the ABC scale. The balance training group scored significantly better than the control group on the BBS ($P < 0.01$) and BESTest ($P < 0.01$). However, no notable variations between groups were observed in the score changes on the ABC scale ($P = 0.2$).

Tai Chi has been shown to be more effective than other usual plan of care therapies for improving balance in patients with COPD. Tai Chi is a form of physical activity characterized by gentle, slow movements, extended periods of standing on one leg, frequent shifts in body weight from side to side and front to back, and contractions of the leg muscles in both lengthening and shortening directions. In individuals without health issues, these actions boost the strength of leg muscles, enhance the sense of joint positioning in the knees and ankles, decrease swaying when standing, and improve the ability to react swiftly to changes in posture, potentially lowering the likelihood of falling. The importance of Tai-chi has been determined by two systematic reviews done by Leung et al. [41] (on 3 RCTs in 2013) and by Ngai et al. [42] (on 12 RCTs in 2016). Meta-analysis of extracted and requested data from authors of original RCTs were done by Review Managing Software in Ngai et al.'s review, whereas, no quantitative analysis were done in the other mentioned review. Both of these reviews compared and contrasted studies incorporating comparisons between utilization of Tai-chi and usual balance exercises programs in addition to pulmonary rehabilitation especially designed for COPD people [41–43].

8. Conclusion

Individuals with COPD face an increased susceptibility to balance issues, underscoring the importance of proactive intervention. Beyond merely attributing this vulnerability to age, we must recognize the profound impact of faulty postures and diminished endurance, consequences of altered respiratory muscle recruitment, and reduced oxygen levels. To navigate the challenges of COPD effectively, it is imperative to integrate a meticulous balance assessment into the foundation of any pulmonary rehabilitation plan. In the realm of COPD management, the incorporation of dynamic evaluations such as the TUG test, SLS, BBS, 6-minute walk test, and ABC questionnaires is not just advisable but crucial. These assessments serve as the compass guiding us toward targeted, personalized interventions that can genuinely transform the landscape of balance for individuals with COPD. Let us not merely acknowledge the hurdles but, more importantly, champion the potential for improvement. Embracing a multifaceted approach that includes static balance training, the meditative grace of Tai-Chi, purposeful transitional exercises, a robust strengthening program, and functional training exercises, we embark on a journey toward enhanced balance and restored vitality for those grappling with COPD. In cultivating a proactive mindset and implementing these tailored strategies, we empower individuals with COPD to reclaim not just physical equilibrium but a renewed sense of control and confidence in their daily lives. By prioritizing and addressing balance challenges head-on, we not only enhance their immediate well-being but also pave the way for a future marked by resilience, strength, and an improved quality of life.

Author details

Qurat Ul Ain[1*], Yasha Sajjad[2] and Tahzeem Riaz[1]

1 Riphah International University, Lahore, Pakistan

2 School of Allied Health Sciences, Combined Military Hospital, Lahore Medical College and Institute of Dentistry, Lahore, Pakistan

*Address all correspondence to: qurat.ain@riphah.edu.pk

References

[1] Gut-Gobert C, Cavaillès A, Dixmier A, Guillot S, Jouneau S, Leroyer C, et al. Women and COPD: Do we need more evidence? European Respiratory Review. 2019;**28**(151):1-13

[2] Holland AE, Cox NS, Houchen-Wolloff L, Rochester CL, Garvey C, ZuWallack R, et al. Defining modern pulmonary rehabilitation. An official American thoracic society workshop report. Annals of the American Thoracic Society. 2021;**18**(5):e12-e29

[3] Vogiatzis I, Rochester CL, Spruit MA, Troosters T, Clini EM. Increasing implementation and delivery of pulmonary rehabilitation: Key messages from the new ATS/ERS policy statement. European Respiratory Journal. 2016;**47**:1336-1341

[4] Oliveira CC, Lee AL, McGinley J, Anderson GP, Clark RA, Thompson M, et al. Balance and falls in acute exacerbation of chronic obstructive pulmonary disease: A prospective study. COPD: Journal of Chronic Obstructive Pulmonary Disease. 2017;**14**(5):518-525

[5] Smith MD, Chang AT, Seale HE, Walsh JR, Hodges PW. Balance is impaired in people with chronic obstructive pulmonary disease. Gait & Posture. 2010;**31**(4):456-460

[6] Garvey C, Novitch RS, Porte P, Casaburi R. Healing pulmonary rehabilitation in the United States. A call to action for ATS members. American Thoracic Society. 2019;**199**:944-946

[7] Kisner C, Colby LA, Borstad J. Therapeutic Exercise: Foundations and Techniques. Philadelphia, United States of America: F.A. Davis Company; 2017

[8] Beauchamp MK. Balance assessment in people with COPD: An evidence-based guide. Chronic Respiratory Disease. 2018;**16**:1479973118820311

[9] Clinic C. Berg balance scale. 2021 [Accessed: Nov 17, 2021]; [cited 2023]. Available from: https://my.clevelandclinic.org/health/diagnostics/22090-berg-balance-scale

[10] Mini balance evaluation systems test. 2013 [cited 2023]. Available from: https://www.sralab.org/rehabilitation-measures/mini-balance-evaluation-systems-test

[11] Albarrati AM, Gale NS, Enright S, Munnery MM, Cockcroft JR, Shale DJ. A simple and rapid test of physical performance in chronic obstructive pulmonary disease. International Journal of Chronic Obstructive Pulmonary Disease. 2016;**11**:1785-1791

[12] Albarrati AM, Gale NS, Munnery MM, Reid N, Cockcroft JR, Shale DJ. The timed up and go test predicts frailty in patients with COPD. NPJ Primary Care Respiratory Medicine. 2022;**32**(1):24

[13] Al Haddad MA, John M, Hussain S, Bolton CE. Role of the timed up and go test in patients with chronic obstructive pulmonary disease. Journal of Cardiopulmonary Rehabilitation and Prevention. 2016;**36**(1):49-55

[14] McLay R, Kirkwood RN, Kuspinar A, Richardson J, Wald J, Raghavan N, et al. Validity of balance and mobility screening tests for assessing fall risk in COPD. Chronic Respiratory Disease. 2020;**17**:1479973120922538

[15] Single leg stance or "One-legged stance test". 2013 [cited 2023].

Available from: https://www.sralab.org/rehabilitation-measures/single-leg-stance-or-one-legged-stance-test

[16] Romberg test. 2013 [cited 2023]. Available from: https://www.sralab.org/rehabilitation-measures/romberg-test

[17] Agrawal Y, Carey JP, Hoffman HJ, Sklare DA, Schubert MC. The modified Romberg balance test: Normative data in US adults. Otology & Neurotology: Official Publication of the American Otological Society, American Neurotology Society [and] European Academy of Otology and Neurotology. 2011;**32**(8):1309

[18] Moreira ACSDS, Mazo GZ, Vieira MP, Machado DB, Cardoso FL, Carvalho RVCD, et al. Evaluating the psychometric properties of the iconographical falls efficacy scale (ICON-FES). Clinics. 2020;**75**:e1427

[19] 6 Minute walk test. 2013 [cited 2023]. Available from: https://www.sralab.org/rehabilitation-measures/6-minute-walk-test

[20] Blennerhassett JM, Dite W, Ramage ER, Richmond ME. Changes in balance and walking from stroke rehabilitation to the community: A follow-up observational study. Archives of Physical Medicine and Rehabilitation. 2012;**93**(10):1782-1787

[21] Activities-specific balance confidence scale [cited 2023]. Jan 2022. Available from: https://www.physio-pedia.com/Activities-Specific_Balance_Confidence_Scale

[22] Mooyeon Oh-Park M, Deepthi Ganta MD. Assessment and treatment of balance impairments. 2016. [updated 2021; cited 2023]. Available from: https://now.aapmr.org/assessment-and-treatment-of-balance-impairments/

[23] Zahra S, Waris M, Ain QU, Sajjad Y. Normative data of modified Romberg balance test for risk of fall in elderly population of Pakistan. JPMA The Journal of the Pakistan Medical Association. 2023;**73**(3):515-519

[24] Khan N, Nasir S, Saeed A, Riaz H. Normative data of balance error in young females. Rawal Medical Journal. 2021;**46**(2):426

[25] Lawlor DA, Patel R, Ebrahim S. Association between falls in elderly women and chronic diseases and drug use: Cross sectional study. BMJ. 2003;**327**(7417):712-717

[26] Beauchamp M, Hill K, Goldstein R, Janaudis-Ferreira T, Brooks D. Impairments in balance discriminate fallers from non-fallers in COPD. Respiratory Medicine. 2009;**103**(12):1885-1891

[27] Tinetti ME, Speechley M, Ginter SF. Risk factors for falls among elderly persons living in the community. New England Journal of Medicine. 1988;**319**(26):1701-1707

[28] Gephine S, Mucci P, Grosbois J-M, Maltais F, Saey D. Physical frailty in COPD patients with chronic respiratory failure. International Journal of Chronic Obstructive Pulmonary Disease. 2021;**16**:1381-1392

[29] Rochester CL, Singh SJ. Increasing Pulmonary Rehabilitation Uptake after Hospitalization for Chronic Obstructive Pulmonary Disease Exacerbation. Let's Rise to the Challenge. New York, United States of America: American Thoracic Society; 2020. pp. 1464-1466

[30] Miravitlles M, Ribera A. Understanding the impact of symptoms on the burden of COPD. Respiratory Research. 2017;**18**(1):1-11

[31] Massierer D, Alsowayan W, Lima VP, Bourbeau J, Janaudis-Ferreira T. Prognostic value of simple measures of physical function and muscle strength in COPD: A systematic review. Respiratory Medicine. 2020;**161**:105856

[32] Elbehairy AF, Faisal A, McIsaac H, Domnik NJ, Milne KM, James MD, et al. Mechanisms of orthopnoea in patients with advanced COPD. European Respiratory Journal. 2021;**57**(3):1-12

[33] Liwsrisakun C, Pothirat C, Chaiwong W, Techatawepisarn T, Limsukon A, Bumroongkit C, et al. Diagnostic ability of the timed up & go test for balance impairment prediction in chronic obstructive pulmonary disease. Journal of Thoracic Disease. 2020;**12**(5):2406

[34] Tudorache E, Oancea C, Avram C, Fira-Mladinescu O, Petrescu L, Timar B. Balance impairment and systemic inflammation in chronic obstructive pulmonary disease. International Journal of Chronic Obstructive Pulmonary Disease. 2015;**10**:1847-1852

[35] Brown AP. Reducing falls in elderly people: A review of exercise interventions. Physiotherapy Theory and Practice. 1999;**15**(2):59-68

[36] Chuatrakoon B, Ngai SP, Sungkarat S, Uthaikhup S. Balance impairment and effectiveness of exercise intervention in chronic obstructive pulmonary disease—A systematic review. Archives of Physical Medicine and Rehabilitation. 2020;**101**(9):1590-1602

[37] de Castro LA, Ribeiro LR, Mesquita R, de Carvalho DR, Felcar JM, Merli MF, et al. Static and functional balance in individuals with COPD: Comparison with healthy controls and differences according to sex and disease severity. Respiratory Care. 2016;**61**(11):1488-1496

[38] Oliveira CC, McGinley J, Lee AL, Irving LB, Denehy L. Fear of falling in people with chronic obstructive pulmonary disease. Respiratory Medicine. 2015;**109**(4):483-489

[39] Riaz T, Ul Ain Q, Amjad M. Comparison of balance impairment among chronic obstructive pulmonary disease (COPD) and healthy population. PJMHS. 2022;**16**(1):659-662

[40] Sampath M. 5 Exercises to improve your balance. 2019 [cited 2023]. Available from: https://www.athletico.com/2019/10/16/5-exercises-to-improve-your-balance/#:~:text=Tandem%20walking%3A&text=Walk%20with%20one%20foot%20in,10%20foot%20length%2C%20four%20times

[41] Leung RW, McKeough ZJ, Alison JA. Tai Chi as a form of exercise training in people with chronic obstructive pulmonary disease. Expert Review of Respiratory Medicine. 2013;7(6):587-592

[42] Ngai SP, Jones AY, San Tam WW. Tai Chi for chronic obstructive pulmonary disease (COPD). Cochrane Database of Systematic Reviews. 2016;(6):1-74

[43] Beauchamp MK, Janaudis-Ferreira T, Parreira V, Romano JM, Woon L, Goldstein RS, et al. A randomized controlled trial of balance training during pulmonary rehabilitation for individuals with COPD. Chest. 2013;**144**(6):1803-1810

Chapter 7

Chronic Obstructive Pulmonary Disease and Gait Disturbance: Is There Any Meaningful Link? Unveiling the Interplay and Addressing the Challenges

Khalid A. Ansari

Abstract

Chronic obstructive pulmonary disease (COPD) is a progressive lung condition characterized by airflow limitation and respiratory symptoms such as shortness of breath, chronic cough, and sputum production. The relationship between COPD and gait disturbance is orchestrated by a complex interplay of factors. Airflow obstruction, the hallmark of COPD, imposes a strain on the respiratory system, leading to breathlessness and fatigue. This relentless struggle for breath forces individuals with COPD to curtail their walking pace, where they adopt a shortened stride and reduced step height. Furthermore, the chronic inflammation associated with COPD infiltrates skeletal muscles, leading to muscle weakness and decreased muscle mass. This insidious process further impairs gait, diminishing the ability to generate the necessary force for efficient ambulation. This chapter will explore the connection between COPD and gait disturbance, examining the underlying mechanisms, prevalence, impact, and management strategies to prevent fall-related injuries and improve the well-being of individuals affected by this challenging combination.

Keywords: COPD, disability, assessment, gait impairment, pulmonary rehabilitation

1. Introduction

The intricate dance between chronic obstructive pulmonary disease (COPD) and gait disturbance is orchestrated by a complex interplay of factors. Airflow obstruction, the hallmark of COPD, imposes a relentless strain on the respiratory system, leading to breathlessness and fatigue. This relentless struggle for breath forces individuals with COPD to curtail their walking pace, where they adopt a shortened stride and reduced step height. Furthermore, the chronic inflammation associated with COPD infiltrates skeletal muscles, leading to muscle weakness and decreased muscle mass. This insidious process further impairs gait, diminishing the ability to generate the necessary force for efficient ambulation.

1.1 Prevalence and impact: a widespread affliction and its consequences

Gait disturbance is not a mere footnote in the saga of COPD; it is a prevalent and debilitating manifestation that significantly impacts the lives of individuals affected. Studies have revealed that over 50% of COPD patients experience gait abnormalities, a proportion that escalates with disease severity. This compromised gait not only hinders daily activities but also increases the risk of falls, a major concern among COPD patients, leading to increased healthcare costs and reduced quality of life.

Current research shows that COPD must be considered as a multidimensional condition [1] with side effects that extend well beyond the lungs. **Figure 1** demonstrates the systemic manifestations of COPD and health outcomes. It begins with the three primary causes of COPD, which include the airway obstruction due to mucus overproduction, airflow limitation, lung hyperinflation, and gas trapping. Lung hyperinflation occurs when trapped air in the lungs makes full exhalation difficult, causes dyspnea, and increases work of breathing (WOB). The dyspnea and WOB, in turn, lead to exercise intolerance. Exercise intolerance is the inability to perform physical activity due to shortness of breath. The lack of exercise can then lead to inactivity and muscle deconditioning, which is the loss of muscle mass and strength, particularly the peripheral muscles, which further could result in frequent hospitalization due to exacerbation, impaired health status, disability, and premature death [2].

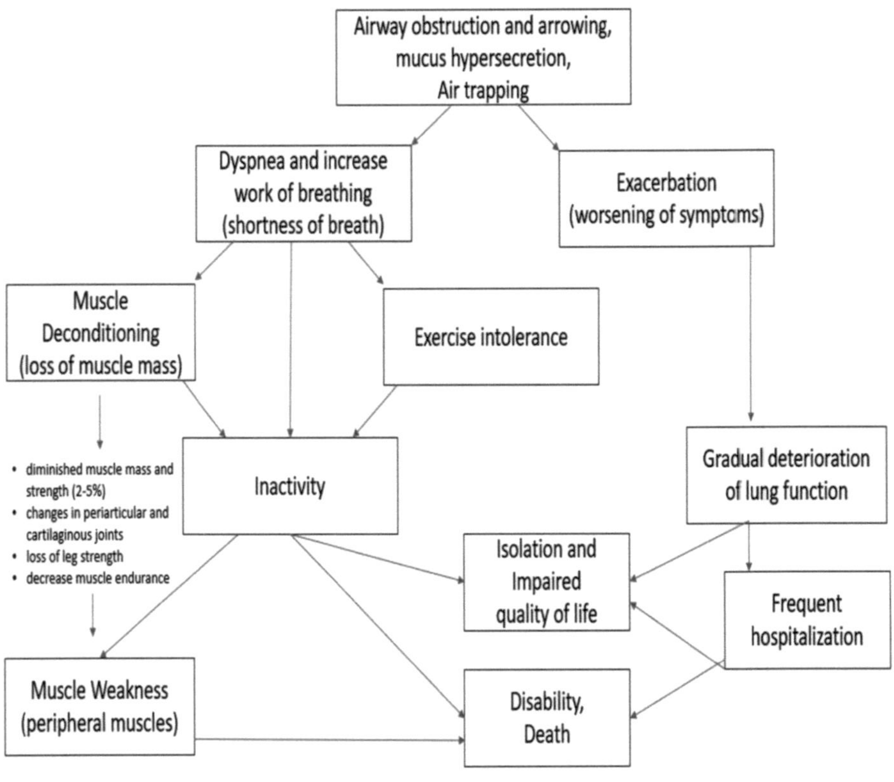

Figure 1.
Consequences of airway obstruction in chronic obstructive pulmonary disease.

DOI: http://dx.doi.org/10.5772/intechopen.1004198

To alleviate this burden, the use of technology for health is being recognized as a tool to identify unseen problems and to provide a potentially effective solution for improving care [3].

People with COPD have a range of characteristics and severity. Therefore, it is fundamental to identify high-risk groups who are likely to suffer from multisystem diseases such as arthritis, osteoporosis, diabetes, and cardiovascular instability [4]. This approach would help to develop early interventions in order to achieve meaningful improvement in their health outcomes. Among many symptoms related to COPD, patients also reported extrapulmonary symptoms, such as coordination and balance issues [5].

Thus, it is essential to improve our understanding about the gait disturbances in COPD and strengthen the gait and balance monitoring systems for COPD with robust technology and customized tools. These personalized tools allow these patients to remain independent, seek medical assistance promptly, and prevent chances of complications such as muscle deconditioning, the risk of fall, and subsequent hospitalizations [6].

1.2 Brief overview of COPD and its prevalence

COPD is characterized by persistent airflow limitation in the lungs. It primarily affects the airways and lung tissues, making it difficult for individuals with COPD to breathe properly [7]. The two main pathological forms of COPD are chronic bronchitis and emphysema, although many patients may have a combination of both conditions [8].

COPD is a significant global health issue and one of the leading causes of morbidity and mortality worldwide [9]. According to the World Health Organization (WHO), as of 2021, it was estimated that more than 250 million people suffer from COPD worldwide [10].

It is estimated that there has been a 27% increase in the number of COPD cases within the last 10 years in the UK. Before the COVID pandemic, the direct cost of COPD to the UK's healthcare system has been estimated at approximately £850 m per annum. The most accurate estimate for the prevalence of diagnosed COPD in England in 2019 among individuals aged 40 years or older is 4.9%. Applying these definitions to the entire population of England using the 2019 mid-year population estimate from the Office of National Statistics suggests that approximately 1.4 million people aged 40 years or older in England have a COPD diagnosis, and an estimated 500,000 are undiagnosed [11].

COPD is a prevalent chronic respiratory disease with substantial global impact. Early diagnosis, prompt intervention, and appropriate management are imperative in improving the quality of life for individuals living with COPD and reducing the burden of this condition on individuals and healthcare systems. Smoking cessation and preventive measures to reduce exposure to risk factors remain essential in curbing both prevalence and complication and/or coexisting conditions, such as gait disturbances.

1.3 Definition and types of gait disturbance

Normal gait is a rhythmic and coordinated pattern of movement that allows humans to walk efficiently and maintain balance. It is characterized by several key features. **Figure 2** shows the different phases of the normal gait cycle in humans.

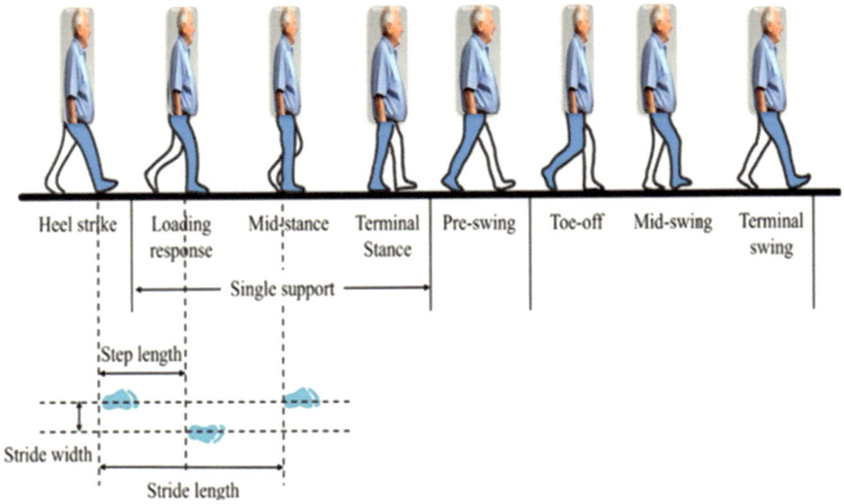

Figure 2.
Phases of a normal gait cycle. Source [12].

The gait cycle is the sequence of events that occurs during one step. It is divided into two main phases: stance phase and swing phase and has several key features, mainly symmetry, stability, efficiency, and smoothness. Firstly, both legs move in a similar manner, with equal stride length and swing time known as symmetry [12]. Stability means that the center of gravity remains relatively stable throughout the gait cycle, minimizing the risk of falls. Efficiency occurs when the muscles work together in a coordinated manner to generate the necessary force for propulsion with minimal energy expenditure. Smoothness refers to a smooth and effortless motion free of jerky or awkward motions [13].

Gait disturbance refers to abnormal walking patterns or difficulties in maintaining a stable and coordinated gait. It is a common issue observed in various medical conditions, affecting mobility, balance, and overall functional abilities [14]. Gait disturbances can vary in severity and presentation, depending on the underlying cause. Gait speed, chair rise time, and the ability to tandem walk are independent predictors of the ability to do daily and instrumental activities of living and of the risk of nursing home admission and death [15].

2. Connections between COPD and gait disturbance

2.1 Prevalence and risk factors for gait disturbance in COPD patients

Consistent evidence shows gait disturbances among people with COPD [16–18]. The prevalence of gait disturbances in COPD patients depends on the severity of the disease, the presence of comorbidities, and the age of the individual. Studies have reported that gait disturbances can affect up to 60% of COPD patients, particularly those with more advanced disease stages [19].

Several risk factors cause gait impairments in people with COPD both directly related to the underlying lung condition and indirectly associated with the age, drugs, lifestyle, and overall health status of the individual [20].

However, the key risk factor that may disrupt balance is muscle weakness. COPD is associated with muscle wasting and weakness, especially in the respiratory muscles and the lower extremities. Weak leg muscles can significantly impact gait stability and lead to walking difficulties [21, 22].

Another potential factor is a reduced exercise capacity. COPD patients often experience exercise intolerance due to impaired lung function, which leads to reduced physical activity [23]. Lack of regular exercise can contribute to deconditioning and further exacerbate gait disturbances.

In addition, breathlessness, which is a hallmark symptom of COPD, particularly individuals with severe dyspnea (shortness of breath), may lead the patient to adopt altered gait patterns to minimize exertion and oxygen demand [24].

Another potential factor is that COPD patients may experience balance problems caused by either muscle weakness or impaired proprioception (sense of body position) [25]. Balance issues can lead to an unsteady gait and an increased risk of falls [26]. In addition, some medications used to control symptoms in COPD, such as bronchodilators or systemic corticosteroids secondary to musculoskeletal abnormalities, can cause muscle weakness or dizziness, which may, in turn, lead to gait-related issues [27–29].

Furthermore, COPD is associated with other chronic conditions and/or complications, such as cardiovascular diseases, osteoporosis, and neurological disorders, which can contribute to gait disturbances [30]. Another integral factor that could be related to balance impairment is smoking, which is a significant risk factor for COPD development [31]. Smoking is known to have an impact on vascular health and contribute to peripheral artery disease or nerve damage, affecting gait [32].

Additionally, unhealthy lifestyle habits and a lack of physical activity can further exacerbate gait issues [33]. Also, COPD is more prevalent in older individuals and age-related changes in muscle strength, joint flexibility, and balance can contribute to gait disturbances in this population [34]. Moreover, COPD patients usually have a range of severity from mild to moderate and severe that causes respiratory muscle weakness and deconditioning, which can influence gait patterns [35].

Therefore, understanding the risk factors for gait disturbance in COPD patients is essential for healthcare professionals to develop appropriate management strategies. Pulmonary rehabilitation, which includes exercise training, can help improve muscle strength and exercise tolerance, leading to better gait stability. Additionally, fall risk assessments and interventions to improve balance can help reduce the risk of falls in COPD patients with gait disturbances.

2.2 Impact of gait disturbance in patients with COPD

2.2.1 Physical and psychological well-being

The altered walking pattern and reduced mobility can affect various aspects of a person's life, leading to functional limitations and emotional challenges. Both the physical and psychological well-being are affected, [36] especially for those individuals with various long-term diseases, such as COPD, which is a heterogeneous condition with multiple phenotypes and endotypes [37].

Gait disturbances can hinder a person's ability to move around independently and perform activities of daily living. Thus, the sufferers become partly dependent to perform activities of daily living on their partner, spouse, family, and/or social support agencies. An unsteady gait can significantly increase the risk of falls, particularly in older adults and in those with weakened muscles or balance impairments. Falls can result in injuries, fractures, and hospitalization, leading to a decline in overall physical health [38].

2.2.2 Muscle fatigue and discomfort

Individuals with gait disturbances may experience muscle fatigue and discomfort due to compensatory movements or abnormal weight distribution while walking [39]. This discomfort can lead to increased energy expenditure and decreased endurance during walking. In patients with COPD, gait disturbances can aggravate breathing difficulties [40].

The additional physical effort required to walk can exacerbate dyspnea, leading to reduced exercise tolerance and further limitations in physical activities [41].

2.2.3 Impact on psychological well-being

Gait disturbances can lead to a loss of independence and to a sense of reliance on others for care and daily tasks [42]. This loss of autonomy can result in feelings of frustration, helplessness, and low self-esteem [43].

Furthermore, anxiety and fear of falling are higher in individuals with gait disturbances, which can be debilitating and lead to social isolation and limitation of their activities that require standing and/or walking such as bathing, walking, exercising, and shopping. This fear of falling may discourage individuals from engaging in physical activities and social interactions [44].

2.2.3.1 Depression and social isolation

The limitations imposed by gait disturbances in people with chronic conditions, such as COPD, can lead to feelings of sadness, hopelessness, and depression [45]. Moreover, social isolation is another adverse consequence of balance and gait impairment that may well cause feelings of loneliness and further exacerbate emotional distress [46].

2.2.3.2 Reduced quality of life

The combination of physical limitations and emotional challenges can significantly reduce the overall quality of life for individuals with gait disturbances. Their ability to engage in meaningful activities and enjoy life may be compromised [46].

Therefore, recognizing the impact of gait disturbance on physical and psychological well-being is essential in developing comprehensive care plans for affected individuals.

Multidisciplinary approaches, including physical therapy, pulmonary rehabilitation, and psychological support, can help improve mobility, manage anxiety and depression, and enhance overall well-being. Providing assistive devices and mobility aids can also promote independence and reduce the risk of falls, enabling individuals to maintain an active and fulfilling lifestyle despite gait disturbances.

2.3 Mechanisms linking COPD to gait disturbance

The mechanisms linking COPD to gait disturbance involve a combination of respiratory and musculoskeletal factors that include airflow limitation, dyspnea, hyperinflation, exacerbation, smoking, steroid use, and respiratory muscle weakness [47].

2.3.1 Airflow limitation

COPD causes chronic airflow limitation, leading to increased work of breathing. The respiratory muscles, including the diaphragm and intercostal muscles, weaken due to the constant effort required to overcome airflow obstruction. This weakness affects breathing during physical activities, such as walking [48].

2.3.2 Dyspnea

COPD patients may experience breathlessness while walking, altering breathing patterns and potentially affecting consistently lower body oxygen and higher carbon dioxide levels, which may lead to altered blood pH, muscle tissue destruction, and muscle weakness. The effect on muscles could be one of the risk factors for balance impairments in this cohort [49].

2.3.3 Muscle wasting, weakness, and deconditioning

Chronic inflammation in COPD can cause muscles, including those involved in walking, to waste, and lose muscle mass. Lower limb muscle weakness affects gait stability and body weight support [50]. Reduced exercise capacity and physical activity limitations in COPD lead to deconditioning, further exacerbating muscle weakness, endurance, and gait abnormalities [51].

2.3.4 Reduced exercise capacity

The combination of impaired lung function and respiratory muscle weakness significantly reduces exercise capacity and tolerance in COPD patients. Exercise capacity refers to the maximum amount of work a person can perform before becoming fatigued. Exercise tolerance, on the other hand, refers to the ability to sustain physical activity for a prolonged period. The reduced exercise capacity and tolerance may lead to compensatory mechanisms during walking, such as slower pace or avoiding strenuous activities [52].

2.3.5 Decreased ventilation-perfusion matching

Ventilation-perfusion (V/Q) mismatch is a major contributing factor to COPD pathology. With V/Q mismatch, the blood in the capillaries does not receive enough oxygen from the air in the alveoli. This oxygen-deprived blood then travels to the muscles, where it cannot provide the necessary oxygen for muscle contraction. As a result, the muscles become weak and fatigued, which can lead to gait impairment. COPD leads to uneven distribution of ventilation and blood flow in the lungs, affecting gas exchange. This can reduce oxygen delivery to muscles during physical activities, impacting gait [53, 54].

2.3.6 Reduced proprioception

COPD patients may experience balance issues, resulting from reduced proprioception, vestibular dysfunction, or musculoskeletal limitations. These impairments contribute to an unsteady gait and increase fall risk [55].

COPD is a progressive lung disease that can significantly impact mobility and increase the risk of falls. One of the key factors contributing to gait disturbances and falls in COPD patients is balance dysfunction. Balance is a complex process that involves the integration of sensory information from the visual, vestibular, and proprioceptive systems along with the coordinated action of the musculoskeletal system.

Reduced proprioception is a common impairment in COPD patients. This sensory deficit can arise from damage to sensory receptors in the muscles, joints, and tendons, often as a result of chronic inflammation and deconditioning associated with COPD. When proprioception is impaired, individuals have difficulty perceiving their body's position and movement in space, making it challenging to maintain balance and stability during walking or standing.

Vestibular dysfunction, another contributing factor to balance issues in COPD patients, originates from abnormalities in the inner ear, which plays a vital role in regulating balance and spatial orientation. Vestibular dysfunction can manifest as dizziness, vertigo, or a sense of unsteadiness, further compounding the challenges of maintaining balance during ambulation.

2.3.7 Medication side effects

Medications used to treat COPD can sometimes cause gait impairment and balance issues. These issues occur because some COPD medications, such as beta-blockers and corticosteroids, can have side effects that affect the muscles and nerves involved in movement [56]. These side effects can include weakness, muscle wasting, and muscle cramps. As a result, people with COPD who are taking these medications may experience difficulty walking, balance problems, and an increased risk of falls.

It is important to note that not all people with COPD will experience gait impairment or balance issues caused by their medication. The risk of these side effects is also increased by other factors such as age, smoking history, and underlying medical conditions. Patients concerned about gait impairment or balance issues should talk to their doctor, who can help to identify whether a medication is causing these problems and can recommend alternative treatment options or additional interventions, such as physical therapy, to help improve mobility.

2.3.8 Coexisting comorbidities

COPD often coexists with other conditions, such as cardiovascular diseases or neurological disorders, which can influence gait mechanics and contribute to gait disturbances.

Some of the most common comorbidities that can contribute to balance impairment in COPD include heart disease, neuromuscular disorders, arthritis, and osteoporosis. Heart disease and stroke can both affect balance by reducing blood flow to the brain and inner ear. Neuromuscular diseases, such as Parkinson's disease and multiple sclerosis, can damage the nerves and muscles that control balance.

Arthritis can cause pain and stiffness in the joints, which can make it difficult to move and maintain balance. Diabetes can damage the nerves and blood vessels in the feet, which can lead to balance problems. Osteoporosis is a condition that weakens the bones, which can make them more likely to break in a fall [56].

Regular assessment and effective management of comorbidities, combined with targeted interventions, can significantly improve gait function and overall quality of life in COPD patients.

2.3.9 Systemic inflammation

COPD's chronic inflammatory state can have systemic effects on muscle function and overall physical performance. Studies have shown a strong correlation between the severity of systemic inflammation in COPD patients and the degree of balance impairment [57]. Patients with higher levels of inflammatory biomarkers exhibit poorer performance on balance tests and a higher risk of falls.

Therefore, systemic inflammation is associated with gait disturbances in individuals with COPD, impacting mobility, balance, and overall functional abilities. Addressing these factors through pulmonary rehabilitation, physical therapy, and targeted interventions can help improve gait and overall quality of life for affected individuals.

Therefore, it is an unmet need to address systemic inflammation in COPD patients, and it may be a good strategy for improving balance function and reducing the risk of falls. Anti-inflammatory medications, such as corticosteroids, have shown some benefit in improving balance in COPD patients [58]. Additionally, lifestyle modifications, such as smoking cessation, regular exercise, and weight management, can help reduce systemic inflammation and potentially improve balance.

2.4 Explanation of gait disturbance and its significance in COPD patients

A growing body of evidence shows that individuals with COPD have critical deficits in balance control that may be associated with gait disturbances and increased risk of falls. The studies reported a fall rate of up to 50% in this population. The presence of balance deficits and gait disturbances has been identified as a significant risk factor for falls in COPD patients [59–62]. Furthermore, the long-term alteration of posture (breathing at a high lung volume [hyperinflated lungs], which causes a slight backward displacement of the thorax and high shoulder position), muscle dysfunction, and the use of steroids, may lead to breathing and gait disturbances [12, 63]. The current findings suggest that COPD patients, in most severe cases, walk less than 15 minutes per day [5].

Moreover, COPD patients walk slower than other people of the same age and have a higher incidence of falls per 1000 people compared with non-COPD subjects. The incidence was 44.9 per 1000 person-years (95% CI 44.1–45.8) for COPD subjects and 24.1 per 1000 person-years (95% CI 23.8–24.5) for non-COPD subjects [16].

COPD cohorts are identified by a range of features, such as a barrel-shaped chest caused by hyperinflation, as shown in **Figure 3**. A barrel-shaped chest, also known as a hyperinflated chest, is a common symptom of COPD. It results from the trapping of air in the lungs due to narrowed airways and damaged alveoli [64]. This air trapping can lead to several anatomical and physiological changes that contribute to gait disturbances in COPD patients.

Other factors, including severity of disease and lifestyle limitations, are important to understand and explore to prevent gait disturbances. Early intervention to mitigate these disturbances can also improve health outcomes. Thus, it is important to strengthen the monitoring systems using robust technology to evaluate their extrapulmonary manifestations and develop technology-centered models and tools that allow these patients to remain independent, motivated, and stable to avoid complications, such as decompensation and hospitalizations.

In addition, COPD people showed a statistically significant reduction, compared to controls, in the stiffness coefficient and viscous damping of the knee joint, as

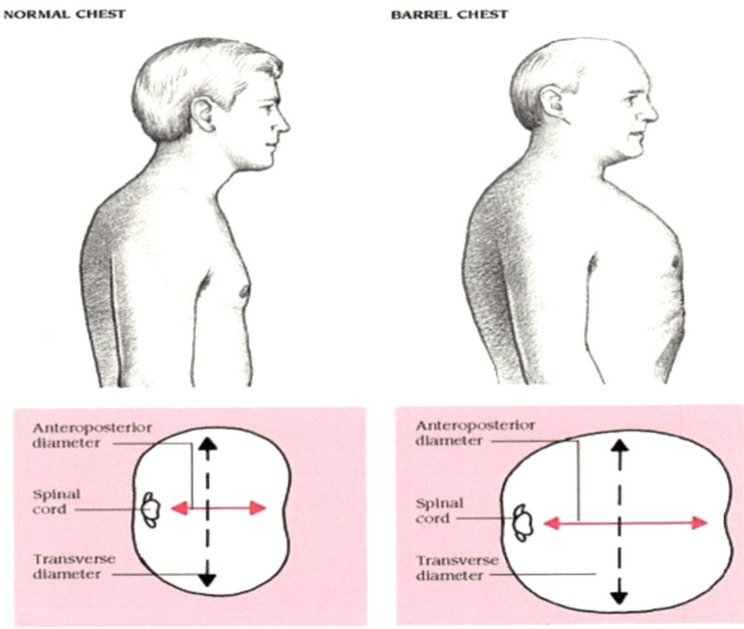

Figure 3.
A normal and a barrel-shaped chest.

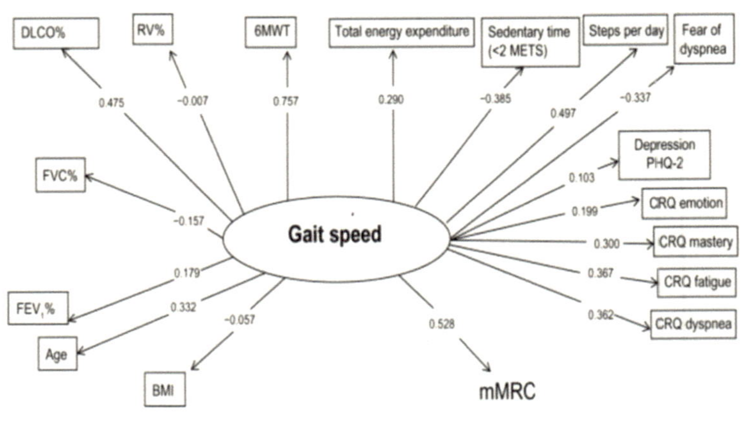

Gait speed construct: correlation (*r*) between psychological and functional variables.

Abbreviations: 6MWT, 6-minute walk test; BMI, body mass index; CRQ, chronic respiratory questionnaire; DLCO, diffusing capacity of the lung for carbon monoxide; FEV_1, forced expiratory volume in one second; FVC, forced vital capacity; METS, metabolic equivalent task; mMRC, modified Medical Research Council; PHQ-2, patient health questionnaire-2; RV, residual volume.

Figure 4.
The relationship of gait speed with physiological parameters in COPD [16].

determined from experiments where the leg is allowed to swing freely after being released from a given angle [65, 66]. These measurements indicate degeneration of the knee tissues. During voluntary flexion-extension movements, electromyography recordings revealed lower activity in the rectus femoris and biceps femoris muscles of COPD patients compared to controls. This reduced muscle activity, likely due to the low viscoelastic tension observed in the patients, contributed to impaired movement performance. These findings offer new perspectives on the underlying mechanisms responsible for movement limitations associated with COPD. Also, Karmpan and co-workers [16] found gait speed as a measure of functional status in COPD individuals is strongly correlated with disease outcomes (**Figure 4**). The arrows in the diagram indicate the direction of the associations. For example, the arrow from lung function to gait speed indicates that people with poor lung function have slower gait speed. This also highlights the fact that exercise capacity is not only the primary determinant of gait speed but also reflects a broader picture of health in COPD patients.

It is important to note that the associations between gait speed and the other variables in the diagram are complex and can be influenced by a number of other factors such as medication use, comorbidities, and lifestyle choices. This complexity arises because it encompasses the interplay of various systems affected by disease severity rather than just lung function alone. As a result, gait speed serves as a valuable screening tool for both exercise capacity and frailty.

In COPD, the usual gait speed measured over a 4-meter course with a rolling start accurately identifies clinically meaningful benchmarks of the 6-minute walk test. Notably, a specific cut-off point of 0.8 m/s has a high positive predictive value (69%) for identifying very poor exercise capacity and an even higher negative predictive value (98%) [67].

The growing body of evidence on gait speed is promising, suggesting its potential as a simple test that comprehensively informs clinicians about various functional aspects of a COPD patient's health. Future research is likely to further demonstrate its strength as a predictive marker for hospitalizations, readmissions, and even mortality.

However, the current assessments of COPD, which are mainly focused on improving symptoms and monitoring disease, do not fully reflect the multisystem impact of the disease. It is, therefore, a vital prerequisite to adapt a holistic approach to managing people with COPD such as promoting physical activity with a higher level of acceptability and mobility that is safe, effective, reliable, and prevents the risk of fall.

Therefore, the functional gait assessment (FGA) to assess postural stability and balance during pulmonary rehabilitation (PR) in COPD populations would identify abnormalities and sensorimotor postural deficiencies. This assessment provides clinicians an opportunity to improve health outcomes in the COPD population. Also, the current international guidelines do not include balance training and fall prevention strategies, which, in turn, lead to risk of fall and impaired quality of life. However, due to limited research in this area, small sample sizes, gender differences, and disease severity, there is lack of evidence to understand the mechanistic link found between such gait impairments and falls in patients with COPD. This suggests that it is important for clinicians to be open-minded to understand the extent and type of support needed to cater to people with COPD. PR is a key therapeutic intervention for individuals with COPD. This situation raises the opportunity to use advanced technology to examine the biomechanics in people with COPD and understand the gait-related impairments these patients have as a guide to develop further accurate standardized assessment tools to identify and manage these impairments.

Gait assessment and rehabilitation for COPD patients extend beyond simply physical exercises. Research suggests that incorporating cognitive stimulation into the process can significantly improve overall outcomes [67–69]. This includes factors such as engagement, motivation, and adherence, which play a crucial role in patient performance and progress.

However, social robots are emerging as innovative tools in healthcare, offering promising benefits for COPD patients undergoing gait rehabilitation. Their physical embodiment and capabilities in social and emotional intelligence contribute to a more engaging and cognitively stimulating experience for users [57, 70]. This, in turn, leads to improved user engagement, task performance, motivation, and ultimately, adherence to the rehabilitation program [19, 71].

The integration of social robots in rehabilitation can have benefits and distinct advantages. One advantage is one-on-one support; social robots provide personalized support, enabling healthcare professionals to dedicate more time and attention to individual patient needs [59]. Also, robots can be utilized as a tool for gait assessment, complementing traditional methods and providing valuable data for healthcare professionals to analyze and tailor treatment plans accordingly [63].

Furthermore, the engaging and motivating nature of social robots can significantly improve patient adherence to the rehabilitation program, leading to better long-term outcomes, [71] and can provide both physical and cognitive assistance, contributing to improved gait performance and overall well-being [57].

3. Approaches to combat COPD-induced musculoskeletal impairments

Several mechanisms contribute to gait impairments in patients with COPD. These include muscle loss, particularly in the legs, due to decreased physical activity. This loss can lead to instability and difficulty walking. Another cause is breathlessness as almost all COPD patients often experience breathlessness, which can further limit their physical activity and contribute to muscle weakness. Furthermore, changes in the lung mechanics, such as hyperinflation and air trapping within the lungs, can lead to changes in posture and gait. Lastly, the psychological fear these patients have can lead to symptoms, such as cough or shortness of breath, which can lead them to avoid activities and lose confidence to do daily activities independently or without support.

These mechanisms collectively have a significant impact on the quality of life of COPD patients. They can also lead to reduced independence, increased social isolation, and increased risk of falls or other serious injuries. The gait issues can increase healthcare costs through more frequent doctor visits, hospital admissions, and long-term care.

3.1 Therapy-based solutions for COPD-induced gait problems

Potential solutions for COPD-induced gait problems include pulmonary rehabilitation (PR), physical therapy (PT), and occupational therapy (OT). The PR program of exercise, education, and support can help COPD patients improve their lung function, physical activity levels, and level of independence. PT can help COPD patients improve their muscle strength, balance, and coordination. A less common intervention, OT, can help COPD patients learn how to modify their daily activities to make them easier and safer. A potentially more effective support can be provided to COPD patients through assistive devices (e.g., canes, rollers) and robot-aided technology.

3.2 Assistive devices

The most emerging solution is the use of assistive technology. Assistive technology can help COPD patients walk more easily and safely. Assistive technologies that can benefit COPD patients with gait problems include:

- Canes: canes can provide support and stability for COPD patients who are at risk of falls [72].
- Walkers: walkers can provide even more support and stability than canes. They can also be used to carry items, such as groceries or oxygen tanks [73].
- Rollators: rollators are walkers with wheels that allow COPD patients to roll instead of walk. The addition of wheels can be helpful for patients who have difficulty walking due to breathlessness or fatigue [74].
- Electric wheelchairs: electric wheelchairs can be used by COPD patients who are unable to walk at all [75].

3.3 Advantages of robot-aided rehabilitation

Robot-aided rehabilitation: robot-aided rehabilitation is a new and emerging technology that is being used to help COPD patients improve their gait. Robots can provide support, guidance, and feedback to help patients learn to walk again.

Robot-aided rehabilitation has several potential advantages over other forms of rehabilitation. It can provide more consistent and reliable support than is provided by human therapists.

- Robots can be programmed to provide customized exercises for each patient.
- Robots can be used to provide rehabilitation in patients' homes, which can be more convenient and affordable than attending therapy sessions at a clinic.

A recent study showed that robot-aided gait rehabilitation improved gait speed, balance, and quality of life in patients with chronic conditions, such as stroke and Parkinson's [76, 77]. The study also found that robot-aided rehabilitation was more effective than traditional physical therapy.

Overall, evidence is growing that robot-aided rehabilitation is a promising new method to treat gait problems in COPD patients. Further research is needed to determine the long-term benefits of robot-aided rehabilitation and to identify the best ways to use this technology in clinical practice.

The technological developments in the healthcare industry have ameliorated health outcomes in patients with chronic diseases such as COPD by improving their quality of life, promoting independence, and encouraging a self-management approach. The use of technology in the medical field also reduces the hospital burden, which has had a massive impact on many practices of healthcare professionals. Smartphones, tablets, and PCs may help people who have COPD and are living at home as these devices can provide information, education, and guidance on the development of their condition. These technologies can recommend appropriate exercise programs or give advice on how to stop smoking; however, they fail to prove useful for the prevention of musculoskeletal impairments derived from COPD. Further, research is needed to harness the potential of state-of-the-art technology to gain a better understanding of COPD-derived motor impairments and act upon them to improve patients' health condition.

Apart from social encouragement to motivate further exercise, several technologies exist that allow a physical intervention to correct posture and gait patterns.

Diverse exoskeletons have been designed to support daily activities, such as the Wearable Walking Helper [WWH] [78], the McKibben pneumatic muscles orthosis [79], or the exoskeleton for patients and the old [EXPOS] by the Sogang University [80]. Exoskeletons, such as the Ekso GT, improve balance and impact functional status in the recovery of patients with stroke [81].

Assistive devices are also of relevant interest for younger patients with life-long disabilities who wish to complement their locomotion skills. For instance, recent advancements allowed patients with spinal cord injuries to "be walked" within an exoskeleton so that they [re]experience bipedal walking and standing. For example, Ekso [Ekso Bionics, US, formerly eLEGs] [81] allowed subjects to walk, stand up, and sit down. Another example is the ReWalk [82], which enabled people with paraplegia to perform ambulatory functions. Also, the HAL robot was reported to enable a paraplegic patient to walk [83, 84].

Though exoskeletons are becoming popular, with many research institutions and companies developing such devices as Honda [American Honda Motor Co., Inc.] [85]. Few publications refer to their design and control characteristics and to the effects of wearing the device [86, 87]. Moreover, most of these devices have been designed as prototypes, being mostly tested with healthy young people so far, with few being used in the market. More importantly, to my knowledge, there is no literature, and no research has been done in the development or use of these devices to aid patients with COPD.

3.4 Limitations and challenges of robot-aided rehabilitation

While robot-aided rehabilitation could revolutionize the treatment of gait problems in COPD patients, some limitations and challenges need to be addressed:

- Cost: robot-aided rehabilitation systems are expensive [88].
- Availability: robot-aided rehabilitation systems are not yet widely available [89].
- Training: therapists need to be trained on how to use robot-aided rehabilitation systems [90].
- Patient acceptance: some patients may be uncomfortable or resistant to using robot-aided rehabilitation systems [91].

Despite these limitations, robot-aided rehabilitation is a promising new technology that has the potential to improve the lives of COPD patients with gait problems.

4. Conclusion

COPD is a progressive respiratory condition that can significantly impact mobility and increase the risk of falls. Gait disturbances in COPD are characterized by slower walking speed, shorter steps, and increased variability in gait patterns. These changes can be attributed to a combination of factors, including airway obstruction, muscle weakness, dyspnea (breathlessness), and deconditioning.

Gait impairments are a significant and often under-recognized aspect of COPD. This chapter has explored the intricate relationship between this chronic respiratory condition and gait function, highlighting the multifaceted nature of this complex interaction. We have delved into the physiological, biomechanical, and psychological factors that contribute to gait abnormalities in COPD patients, encompassing topics such as exercise capacity, muscle weakness, dyspnea, and anxiety.

The evidence presented underscores the critical role of gait assessment in the comprehensive management of COPD. Early identification and monitoring of gait impairments are compelling for optimizing rehabilitation strategies, reducing fall risk, and improving overall quality of life. Integrating various assessment tools, including functional tests, gait analysis, and potentially, socially assistive robots, can provide valuable insights into individual patient needs and inform personalized interventions.

Emerging technologies, such as wearable sensors and exoskeletons, offer exciting possibilities for further augment gait rehabilitation in COPD patients. These tools can provide real-time feedback, facilitate targeted interventions, and track progress objectively, leading to more effective and individualized treatment plans.

Looking beyond the immediate impact on gait, the broader implications of the COPD-gait connection are significant. Gait impairments can affect daily activities, social participation, and mental well-being, leading to a reduced quality of life for COPD patients. By addressing these challenges through comprehensive gait rehabilitation programs, we can empower individuals with COPD to maintain their independence, boost their social engagement, and improve their overall well-being.

Furthermore, in this chapter robot-aided technology has emerged as a promising intervention to prevent fall risk in COPD patients. These technologies offer several advantages, including:

Fall detection and alert systems: wearable sensors or smart home devices can detect falls or near-falls and immediately trigger an alarm, notifying caregivers or emergency services. This prompt intervention can significantly reduce the time spent on the ground, minimizing the risk of serious complications.

Gait and balance assistance: robotic exoskeletons or wearable devices can provide real-time support during ambulation, helping to stabilize gait, improve balance, and reduce the risk of tripping or falling. These devices can be particularly beneficial for patients with severe gait disturbances or those who have experienced recurrent falls.

Rehabilitation and exercise support: robotic-assisted rehabilitation programs can provide personalized and intensive gait and balance training, helping patients regain strength, improve coordination, and strengthen their overall mobility. These programs can be customized to individual patient needs and can be tailored to different stages of COPD progression.

Environmental monitoring and assistance: smart home technology can monitor the patient's environment, such as detecting low lighting or slippery floors, and can trigger appropriate interventions, such as turning on lights or activating fall prevention mats. These proactive measures can help to reduce the risk of falls by addressing potential hazards in the home environment.

Telehealth and remote monitoring: robot-aided technology can facilitate remote monitoring of COPD patients, allowing healthcare providers to assess gait patterns, track progress, and provide personalized support and guidance. This can be particularly beneficial for patients in rural or underserved areas who may have limited access to in-person care.

Psychological support and fall prevention education: robot-assisted technology can provide psychological support and fall prevention education, helping patients to develop coping mechanisms, manage anxiety, and adopt safer movement strategies.

These interventions can, further, enhance fall prevention efforts by addressing psychological factors that may contribute to fall risk.

Integration of robot-aided technology into COPD care may significantly reduce fall risk and improve mobility outcomes for these patients. By providing personalized support, real-time monitoring, and remote intervention capabilities, these technologies can play a crucial role in reviving the quality of life and safety of individuals living with COPD.

By implementing these strategies, healthcare providers and caregivers can effectively support COPD patients with gait and balance issues, improving their mobility, reducing fall risk, and lifting their overall quality of life.

The future holds immense potential for further advancements in understanding and addressing the complex relationship between COPD and gait. Continued research efforts are needed to explore the efficacy of innovative technologies, develop new therapeutic strategies, and improve the overall management of gait impairments in COPD patients. This multifaceted approach is preeminent for ensuring that individuals with COPD can lead active and fulfilling lives.

Author details

Khalid A. Ansari
Faculty of Medical and Health Sciences, Liwa College, Abu Dhabi, UAE

*Address all correspondence to: khalid.ansari@lc.ac.ae

References

[1] Antonelli Incalzi R, Canonica GW, Scichilone N, Rizzoli S, Simoni L, Blasi F, et al. The COPD multi-dimensional phenotype: A new classification from the STORICO Italian observational study. PLoS One. 2019;**14**(9):e0221889. DOI: 10.1371/journal.pone.0221889

[2] Hanania NA, Donohue JF. Pharmacologic interventions in chronic obstructive pulmonary disease: Bronchodilators. Proceedings of the American Thoracic Society. 2007;**4**(7):526-534

[3] Wang Z, Yang Z, Dong T. A review of wearable technologies for elderly care that can accurately track indoor position, recognize physical activities and monitor vital signs in real time. Sensors. 2017;**17**(2):341

[4] Gore S, Blackwood J, Ziccardi T. Associations between cognitive function, balance, and gait speed in community-dwelling older adults with COPD. Journal of Geriatric Physical Therapy. 2023;**46**(1):46-52

[5] McCabe C, McCann M, Brady A. Computer and mobile technology interventions for self-management in chronic obstructive pulmonary disease. Cochrane Database of Systematic Reviews. 2017;**5**:CD011425. DOI: 10.1002/14651858.CD011425.pub2

[6] Arai H, Nozoe M, Kamiya K, Matsumoto S, Morimoto T. Association between skeletal muscle mass index and falls in patients with functional impairment. American Journal of Physical Medicine & Rehabilitation. 2023;**102**(10):913-918

[7] Öztürk BÇ, Gemicioğlu B. Pathophysiology of the upper and lower airways. In: Airway Diseases. Cham: Springer International Publishing; 2023. pp. 1-14

[8] Prasad B. Chronic obstructive pulmonary disease [COPD]. International Journal of Pharmacy Research & Technology [IJPRT]. 2020;**10**(1):67-71

[9] Lortet-Tieulent J, Soerjomataram I, López-Campos JL, Ancochea J, Coebergh JW, Soriano JB. International trends in COPD mortality, 1995-2017. European Respiratory Journal. 2019;**54**(6):1-4

[10] Respiratory disease: Applying All Our Health. GOV.UK. 2022. Available from: https://www.gov.uk/government/publications/respiratory-disease-applying-all-our-health/respiratory-disease-applying-all-our-health

[11] Office for National Statistics. Population Estimates for the UK, England and Wales, Scotland and Northern Ireland; 2019. Available from: https://www.ons.gov.uk/peoplepopulationandcommunity/populationandmigration/populationestimates/bulletins/annualmidyearpopulationestimates/mid2019estimates [Accessed: February 09, 2023]

[12] CorlateanuA,PlahotniucA,CorlateanuO, Botnaru V, Bikov A, Mathioudakis AG, et al. Multidimensional indices in the assessment of chronic obstructive pulmonary disease. Respiratory Medicine. 2021;**185**:106519. DOI: 10.1016/j.rmed.2021.106519. Epub 2021 Jun 22

[13] Lei Y, Yang F. Simulation analysis and study of gait stability related to motion joints. BioMed Research

International. 2022;**2022**:8417089. DOI: 10.1155/2022/8417089

[14] Keogh JW, Senior H, Beller EM, Henwood T. Prevalence and risk factors for low habitual walking speed in nursing home residents: An observational study. Archives of Physical Medicine and Rehabilitation. 2015;**96**(11):1993-1999

[15] Kuys SS, Peel NM, Klein K, Slater A, Hubbard RE. Gait speed in ambulant older people in long term care: A systematic review and meta-analysis. Journal of the American Medical Directors Association. 2014;**15**(3):194

[16] Karpman C, Depew ZS, Lebrasseur NK, Novotny PJ, Benzo RP. Determinants of gait speed in chronic obstructive lung disease. Chest. 2014;**1**:104-110

[17] DePew ZS, Karpman C, Novotny PJ, Benzo RP. Correlations between gait speed, 6-minute walk distance, physical activity, and self-efficacy in patients with severe chronic lung disease. Respiratory Care. 2013;**58**(12):2113-2119

[18] Kon SS, Patel MS, Canavan JL, et al. Reliability and validity of the four metre gait speed in COPD. The European Respiratory Journal. 2012;**12**:2113-2119

[19] Kaygusuz MH, Oral Tapan O, Tapan U, Genc S. Balance impairment and cognitive dysfunction in patients with chronic obstructive pulmonary disease under 65 years. The Clinical Respiratory Journal. 2022;**16**(3):200-207

[20] Marshall FJ. Approach to the elderly patient with gait disturbance. Neurology: Clinical Practice. 2012;**2**(2):103-111

[21] Seymour JM, Spruit MA, Hopkinson NS, Natanek SA, Man WC, Jackson A, et al. The prevalence of quadriceps weakness in COPD and the relationship with disease severity. European Respiratory Journal. 2010;**36**(1):81-88

[22] Polkey MI. Peripheral muscle weakness in COPD: Where does it come from? Thorax. 2003;**58**(9):741-742

[23] Pepin V, Saey D, Laviolette L, Maltais F. Exercise capacity in chronic obstructive pulmonary disease: Mechanisms of limitation. COPD: Journal of Chronic Obstructive Pulmonary Disease. 2007;*4*(3):195-204

[24] Hirjaková Z, Neumannová K, Kimijanová J, Šuttová K, Janura M, Hlavačka F. Breathing changes accompanying balance improvement during biofeedback. Neuroscience Letters. 2017;**651**:30-35

[25] Crişan AF, Oancea C, Timar B, Fira-Mladinescu O, Tudorache V. Balance impairment in patients with COPD. PLoS One. 2015;**10**(3):e0120573

[26] Hakamy A, Bolton CE, Gibson JE, McKeever TM. Risk of fall in patients with COPD. Thorax. 2018;**73**(11):1079-1080

[27] Cott RA, Estrada JC, Lowenthal DT. An uncommon cause of unsteady gait in an elderly gentleman. International Urology and Nephrology. 2001;**33**(4):687

[28] Brosch JR, Sant RV, Golomb MR. Subacute onset of abnormal gait and head drop in a 3-year-old with history of extreme prematurity. Journal of Child Neurology. 2011;**26**(3):373-376

[29] Cielen N, Maes K, Gayan-Ramirez G. Musculoskeletal disorders in chronic obstructive pulmonary disease. BioMed Research International. 2014;**2014**:1-17

[30] Negewo NA, Gibson PG, McDonald VM. COPD and its

comorbidities: Impact, measurement and mechanisms. Respirology. 2015;**20**(8):1160-1171

[31] Riesco JA, Alcázar B, Trigueros JA, Campuzano A, Pérez J, Lorenzo JL. Active smoking and COPD phenotype: Distribution and impact on prognostic factors. International Journal of Chronic Obstructive Pulmonary Disease. 2017;**12**:1989-1999

[32] Kumboyono K, Chomsy IN, Hakim AK, Sujuti H, Hariyanti T, Srihardyastutie A, et al. Detection of vascular inflammation and oxidative stress by cotinine in smokers: Measured through Interleukin-6 and superoxide dismutase. International Journal of General Medicine. 2022:7319-7328

[33] Yamaguchi Y, Greiner C, Lee SC, Ryuno H, Yen HY, Lin CF, et al. Lifestyle factors associated with muscle quality in community-dwelling older people with type 2 diabetes in Japan and Taiwan: A cross-sectional study. Psychogeriatrics. 2022;**22**(5):736-742

[34] Boyer KA, Hayes KL, Umberger BR, Adamczyk PG, Bean JF, Brach JS, et al. Age-related changes in gait biomechanics and their impact on the metabolic cost of walking: Report from a National Institute on Aging workshop. Experimental Gerontology. 2023;**112102**:1-11

[35] Heubel AD, Kabbach EZ, Leonardi NT, Schafauser NS, Kawakami DM, Sentanin AC, et al. Respiratory and peripheral muscle strength influence recovery of exercise capacity after severe exacerbation of COPD? An observational prospective cohort study. Heart & Lung. 2023;**58**:91-97

[36] Feldman R, Schreiber S, Pick CG, Been E. Gait, balance and posture in major mental illnesses: Depression, anxiety and schizophrenia. Austin Medical Sciences. 2020;**5**(1):1-6

[37] Corlateanu A, Mendez Y, Wang Y, Garnica RDJA, Botnaru V, Siafakas N. Chronic obstructive pulmonary disease and phenotypes: A state-of-the-art. Pulmonology. 2020;**26**(2):95-100

[38] Pieruccini-Faria F, Montero-Odasso M, Hausdorff JM. Gait variability and fall risk in older adults: The role of cognitive function. Falls and Cognition in Older Persons: Fundamentals, Assessment and Therapeutic Options. 2020;**1**:107-138

[39] Ghani HA, Justine M, Manaf H. Effects of lower limb muscle fatigue on gait performance and postural control among individuals with Parkinson's disease: A review of literature. Physical Therapy Reviews. 2019;**24**(6):274-279

[40] Terui Y, Iwasawa S, Kikuchi K, Furukawa Y, Suto E, Uemura S, et al. The relationship between gait asymmetry and respiratory function in stroke patients: A pilot study. Open Journal of Therapy and Rehabilitation. 2021;**9**(4):111-122

[41] Elbehairy AF, O'Donnell CD, Abd Elhameed A, Vincent SG, Milne KM, James MD, et al. Low resting diffusion capacity, dyspnea, and exercise intolerance in chronic obstructive pulmonary disease. Journal of Applied Physiology. 2019;**127**(4):1107-1116

[42] Li Y, Lyu Y, Song R. Phase-dependent modulation of muscle activity and intermuscular coupling during walking in patients after stroke. IEEE Transactions on Neural Systems and Rehabilitation Engineering. 2023;**31**:1119-1127

[43] Ahn S, Chung JW, Crouter SE, Lee JA, Lee CE, Anderson JG. Gait and/or balance disturbances associated

with Alzheimer's dementia among older adults with amnestic mild cognitive impairment: A longitudinal observational study. Journal of Advanced Nursing. 2023;**12**:4815-4827

[44] Uhlig M, Prell T. Gait characteristics associated with fear of falling in hospitalized people with Parkinson's disease. Sensors. 2023;**23**(3):1111

[45] Chan LL, Brodie MA, Lord SR. Prediction of incident depression in middle-aged and older adults using digital gait biomarkers extracted from large-scale wrist sensor data. Journal of the American Medical Directors Association. 2023;**24**

[46] Kuang K, Huisingh-Scheetz M, Miller MJ, Waite L, Kotwal AA. The association of gait speed and self-reported difficulty walking with social isolation: A nationally-representative study. Journal of the American Geriatrics Society. 2023

[47] Boz HE, Kiriş AÖ, Koçoğlu K, Çolakoğlu BD, Çakmur R, Akdal G. Balance and gait disturbances and quality of life in patients with idiopathic Parkinson'S disease and progressive supranuclear palsy. Neurological Sciences and Neurophysiology. 2021;**38**(1):45-49. DOI: 10.4103/nsn.nsn_148_20

[48] Avila A, Serrado A, Reig L, Famades A, Maho P. Early presentation of gait disturbance in a steroid-responsive encephalopathy associated with autoimmune thyroiditis. European Journal of Neurology. 2003;**10**(5):601. DOI: 10.1046/j.1468-1331.2003.00667.x

[49] Kocjan J, Gzik-Zroska B, Nowakowska K, Burkacki M, Suchoń S, Michnik R, et al. Impact of diaphragm function parameters on balance maintenance. PLoS One. 2018;**13**(12):e0208697. DOI: 10.1371/journal.pone.0208697

[50] Piazza SJ, Delp SL. The influence of muscles on knee flexion during the swing phase of gait. Journal of Biomechanics. 1996;**29**(6):723-733

[51] Oh GB, Park CS, Cho KH. Immediate effect of weight load on lower limb muscle activity and gait ability in patients with incomplete spinal cord injury during walker gait training. The Journal of Spinal Cord Medicine. 2023;**46**(5):818-824

[52] Mallard J, Hucteau E, Schott R, Trensz P, Pflumio C, Kalish-Weindling M, et al. Early skeletal muscle deconditioning and reduced exercise capacity during [neo] adjuvant chemotherapy in patients with breast cancer. Cancer. 2023;**129**(2):215-225

[53] Abdelrahman MGM, Afify AM, Rahmy AF, Abdelwahab MAM. Effect of Biodex training on balance impairment in patients with chronic obstructive pulmonary disease. Journal of Pharmaceutical Negative Results. 2023:2446-2451

[54] Windham BG, Griswold ME, Ranadive R, Sullivan KJ, Mosley TH, Mielke MM, et al. Relationships of cerebral perfusion with gait speed across systolic blood pressure levels and age: A cohort study. The Journals of Gerontology. Series A, Biological Sciences and Medical Sciences. 2023;**78**(3):514-520. DOI: 10.1093/gerona/glac120

[55] Janssens L, Brumagne S, McConnell AK, Claeys K, Pijnenburg M, Burtin C, et al. Proprioceptive changes impair balance control in individuals with chronic obstructive pulmonary disease. PLoS One. 2013;**8**(3):e57949

[56] Zia A, Kamaruzzaman SB, Tan MP. Polypharmacy and falls in older people: Balancing evidence-based medicine

against falls risk. Postgraduate Medicine. 2015;**127**(3):330-337

[57] Denfeld QE, Turrise S, MacLaughlin EJ, Chang PS, Clair WK, Lewis EF, et al. Preventing and managing falls in adults with cardiovascular disease: A scientific statement from the American heart association. Circulation: Cardiovascular Quality and Outcomes. 2022;**15**(6):e000108

[58] Cazzola M, Hanania NA, Page CP, Matera MG. Novel anti-inflammatory approaches to COPD. International Journal of Chronic Obstructive Pulmonary Disease. 2023:1333-1352

[59] Medina-Mirapeix F, Bernabeu-Mora R, Gacto-Sánchez M, Montilla-Herrador J, Escolar-Reina P, Sánchez-Martínez MP. The prognosis of pre-frail chronic obstructive pulmonary disease patients for hospitalizations and mortality depends on their level of functional physical performance. Chronic Respiratory Disease. 2022;**19**:14799731221119810

[60] Shrikrishna D, Patel BK, Patel JM, Bhavsar MJ. Falls in patients with chronic obstructive pulmonary disease: Prevalence, risk factors, and impact on health. Journal of Family Medicine and Primary Care. 2013;**2**(4):662

[61] Holland AE, Spruit MA, Walke MJ, Hopkinson NS, Rochester CL. The prevalence and risk factors for falls in COPD: A systematic review and meta-analysis. Thorax. 2016;**71**(4):347-354

[62] Lee SH, Hong YJ, Park JH. Balance deficits in chronic obstructive pulmonary disease patients: A systematic review and meta-analysis. International Journal of Rehabilitation and Research. 2020;**43**(1):1-13

[63] Respiratory Disease: Applying All Our Health. GOV.UK. 2022. Available from: https://www.gov.uk/government/publications/respiratory-disease-applying-all-our-health/respiratory-disease-applying-all-our-health

[64] Chung E, Lee SH, Lee HJ, et al. Comparative study of young-old and old-old people using functional evaluation, gait characteristics, and cardiopulmonary metabolic energy consumption. BMC Geriatrics. 2023;**23**:400. DOI: 10.1186/s12877-023-04088-6

[65] MacNaughton. Understanding Barrel Chest with COPD. 2019. Available from: https://copd.net/clinical/barrel-chest

[66] Valle MS, Casabona A, Di Fazio E, et al. Impact of chronic obstructive pulmonary disease on passive viscoelastic components of the musculoarticular system. Scientific Reports. 2021;**1**:18077. DOI: 10.1038/s41598-021-97621-9

[67] Mullins LL, Keller JR, Chaney JM. A systems and social cognitive approach to team functioning in physical rehabilitation settings. Rehabilitation Psychology. 1994;**39**(3):161-178

[68] Fabel K, Kempermann G. Physical activity and the regulation of neurogenesis in the adult and aging brain. Neuromolecular Medicine. 2008;**10**:59-66

[69] Beauchamp MK. Balance assessment in people with COPD: An evidence-based guide. Chronic Respiratory Disease. 2019;**16**:1-8. DOI: 10.1177/1479973118820311

[70] Lahousse L, Ziere G, Verlinden VJ, Zillikens MC, Uitterlinden AG, Rivadeneira F, et al. Risk of frailty in elderly with COPD: A population-based study. The Journals of Gerontology. Series A, Biological Sciences and Medical Sciences. 2016;**71**(5):689-695. DOI: 10.1093/gerona/glv154. Epub 2015 Sep 9

[71] Spruit MA, Singh SJ, Garvey C, et al. An official American thoracic society/European respiratory society statement: Key concepts and advances in pulmonary rehabilitation. American Journal of Respiratory and Critical Care Medicine. 2013;**188**(8):e13-e64

[72] American Academy of Physical Medicine and Rehabilitation. Assistive Technology for Fall Prevention in Older Adults. 2023. Available from: https://www.ncbi.nlm.nih.gov/pmc/articles/PMC10172979/

[73] Mayo Clinic. Fall Prevention & Management For Nurses. 2022. Available from: https://www.mayoclinic.org/about-mayo-clinic/quality/quality-measures/falls-prevention

[74] National Institute on Aging. Caregiving: A Guide for Families and Friends. 2023. Available from: https://www.nia.nih.gov/health/caregiving

[75] National Center for Biotechnology Information. Chronic Obstructive Pulmonary Disease: The Role of Occupational Therapy. 2022. Available from: https://www.otdude.com/ot-practice/occupational-therapy-for-copd-in-acute-care-acute-rehab-snf-home-health/

[76] Lamberti N, Manfredini F, Lissom LO, Lavezzi S, Basaglia N, Straudi S. Beneficial effects of robot-assisted gait training on functional recovery in women after stroke: A cohort study. Medicina. 2021;**57**(11):1200. DOI: 10.3390/medicina57111200

[77] Mustafaoglu R, Erhan B, Yeldan I, Gunduz B, Tarakci E. Does robot-assisted gait training improve mobility, activities of daily living and quality of life in stroke? A single-blinded, randomized controlled trial. Acta Neurologica Belgica. 2020;**120**(2):335-344. DOI: 10.1007/s13760-020-01276-8. Epub 2020 Jan 28

[78] Hirata Y, Iwano T, Kosuge K. Control of wearable walking helper on slope based on integration of acceleration and GRF information. In: 2008 IEEE/RSJ International Conference on Intelligent Robots and Systems. IEEE; 2008. pp. 3731-3736

[79] Uchiyama K, Ito T, Tomori H. Development of endoskeleton type knee joint assist orthosis using McKibben type artificial muscle. Journal of Robotics and Mechatronics. 2022;**34**(2):390-401

[80] Shah SH, Alam MS, Arsalan M, Ul Haq I, Khan SG, Iqbal J. Design and adaptive compliance control of a wearable walk assist device. In 2023 International Conference on Robotics and Automation in Industry (ICRAI). 2023

[81] Høyer E, Opheim A, Jørgensen V. Implementing the exoskeleton Ekso GTTM for gait rehabilitation in a stroke unit–feasibility, functional benefits and patient experiences. Disability and Rehabilitation: Assistive Technology. 2022;**17**(4):473-479

[82] Tamburella F, Lorusso M, Tramontano M, Fadlun S, Masciullo M, Scivoletto G. Overground robotic training effects on walking and secondary health conditions in individuals with spinal cord injury: Systematic review. Journal of Neuroengineering and Rehabilitation. 2022;**19**(1):1-56

[83] Suzuki K, Kawamura Y, Hayashi T, Sakurai T, Hasegawa Y, Sankai Y. Intention-based walking support for paraplegia patient. In: 2005 IEEE International Conference on Systems, Man and Cybernetics. Vol. 3. IEEE; 2005. pp. 2707-2713

[84] Watanabe H, Marushima A, Kawamoto H, Kadone H, Ueno T, Shimizu Y, et al. Intensive gait treatment using a robot suit hybrid assistive limb in acute spinal cord infarction: Report of two cases. The Journal of Spinal Cord Medicine. 2019;**42**(3):395-401

[85] Dayani F, Sadeghei-Naeenei H, Bahrami M, Choopankareh V. Assessment of body work condition by RULA method in a motor vehicle industry in order to design an effective exoskeleton system. Iran Occupational Health. 2012;**8**(4):36-47

[86] Fayolle-Minon I, Calmels P. Effect of wearing a lumbar orthosis on trunk muscles: Study of the muscle strength after 21 days of use on healthy subjects. Joint, Bone, Spine. 2008;**75**(1):58-63

[87] Chang CH, Wang MJJ, Lin SC. Evaluating the effects of wearing gloves and wrist support on hand–arm response while operating an in-line pneumatic screwdriver. International Journal of Industrial Ergonomics. 1999;**24**(5):473-481

[88] Morone G, Paolucci S, Cherubini A, De Angelis D, Venturiero V, Coiro P, et al. Robot-assisted gait training for stroke patients: Current state of the art and perspectives of robotics. Neuropsychiatric Disease and Treatment. 2017:1303-1311

[89] Laszlo C, Munari D, Maggioni S, Knechtle D, Wolf P, De Bon D. Feasibility of an intelligent algorithm based on an assist-as-needed controller for a robot-aided gait trainer (Lokomat) in neurological disorders: A longitudinal pilot study. Brain Sciences. 2023;**13**(4):612

[90] Faulkner J, Wright A, Stone K, Fryer S, Martinelli L, Lambrick D, et al. Effect of home-based, overground robotic-assisted gait training on vascular health in people with chronic stroke. Frontiers in Neurology. 2023;**14**:1093008

[91] Cavallo F, Esposito R, Limosani R, Manzi A, Bevilacqua R, Felici E, et al. Robotic services acceptance in smart environments with older adults: User satisfaction and acceptability study. Journal of Medical Internet Research. 2018;**20**(9):e264

Section 5

Future Directions

Chapter 8

Recent Advances in Chronic Obstructive Pulmonary Disease

Biruk Getahun, Abebe Ayalew Bekel, Dessalegn Demeke Ayalew, Melkamu Demewez Gebeye, Dagnachew Zemene and Erstu Legese Beyene

Abstract

The prevalent respiratory condition known as chronic obstructive pulmonary disease (COPD) is associated with high morbidity and death. Despite being common, COPD is underdiagnosed, and many individuals are not diagnosed until the condition has advanced clinically. The early physiologic and pathobiologic alterations in COPD have been the focus of recent fundamental scientific and clinical research in an effort to improve diagnosis, provide targets for disease-modifying medication, and identify people most likely to benefit from early intervention. Good communication with COPD patients requires humanity, respect, and a people-oriented mindset. The healthcare professional's personal values and views may facilitate or obstruct communication. All facets of healthcare share the ideal "personal specifications" for healthcare providers who treat people with COPD. The number of COPD therapies has increased significantly over the past 20 years because of the development of new oral and inhaled medications and novel surgical and bronchoscopic techniques. According to the Global Initiative for Chronic Obstructive Lung Diseases (GOLD) recommendations, bronchodilators such as long-acting muscarinic antagonists (LAMA) are frequently used as the first line of treatment for most symptomatic COPD patients. Stem cells as potential therapeutic tools can differentiate into several different lung cell types such as the alveolar epithelial cells. Gene therapy offers novel therapeutic options for inherited and acquired diseases by delivering exogenous genetic materials into cells or tissues. This review discusses best practices in COPD prevention, diagnosis, and treatment.

Keywords: early intervention, pulmonary disease, diagnosis, COPD, treatment, lung denervation, gene therapy

1. Introduction

With a high prevalence of over 250 million patients worldwide, chronic obstructive pulmonary disease (COPD) is a chronic lung illness that is frequently extremely disabling. It is currently the third-leading cause of death in the world [1, 2]. According to the most recent definition, COPD is "a common, preventable, and treatable disease that is characterized by persistent respiratory systems and airflow limitation due to airway and/or alveolar abnormalities typically caused by significant exposure to noxious particles or gases" [3]. With smoking being the primary risk factor in high-income nations and indoor cooking and occupational exposures serving as significant risk factors in low-income countries, this exposure can vary substantially [1]. Although COPD manifests varied clinical characteristics in individuals, the classification and staging used by the Global Initiative for Chronic Obstructive Lung Diseases (GOLD) are standard, determined by lung function, symptoms, and exacerbation history. Inflammation has long been acknowledged as a key feature of COPD, contributing to the pathological alterations in the various lung compartments [4]. In addition to hazardous exposures, genetic predisposition is a significant risk factor for COPD. Genetic anomalies together with the type and length of exposures produce the clinical phenotype in COPD [5].

Emphysema and chronic bronchitis, which together make up COPD, are caused by an aberrant inflammatory response in the lungs following exposure to noxious particles or gases, which results in airway blockage and emphysematous alterations [6]. Common COPD symptoms include a persistent cough, an abundance of mucus, air entrapment, dynamic hyperinflation, and shortness of breath after exertion [7]. In fact, COPD has symptoms that extend beyond the lungs, including systemic manifestations like inflammation, and it is frequently linked to other illnesses including cardiovascular disease and metabolic syndrome [5, 7]. Breathing problems and sputum production are common exacerbation symptoms of COPD that are connected to recurrent episodes of increased airway and systemic inflammation [8]. Patients with severe COPD are more likely to experience COPD exacerbations, which have also been linked to bacterial or viral infections [6].

Patients with COPD often engage in less daily physical activity than healthy controls due to their breathing difficulty [9]. Additionally, comorbid conditions like anxiety, depression, osteoporosis, and cardiovascular disease are frequently present in COPD patients, which adversely affect their general health, quality of life (QoL), functional status, and clinical outcomes [10]. The healthcare system is burdened by significant direct and indirect expenditures related to COPD. With early detection, adequate treatment, and management, the effects of COPD on patients and society as a whole can be significantly mitigated.

Recent research on COPD has addressed multiple facets of the disease, including medical aspects but also extending to some of the sociological aspects that can affect the disease's diagnosis and the patient's compliance with recommendations for prevention and treatment. This review will discuss the best practices in COPD prevention, diagnosis, and treatment. It will then describe ongoing research that is directed toward potential future approaches to the disease.

2. Pathophysiology

Chronic airway inflammation causes COPD, which results in the thickening of the airway walls, a rise in mucus production, and ultimately permanent alterations to the structure of the lungs [11]. The breakdown of the lung parenchyma, particularly the walls of the air sacs (alveoli), can cause lung alterations such as emphysema and fibrosis of the tiny airways [6, 11]. Breathlessness, coughing, and increased phlegm production may all be signs of these structural alterations, which can also result in severe air trapping and hyperinflation [7].

Elevated neutrophils, activated macrophages, and activated CD8+ T lymphocytes indicate chronic lung inflammation in COPD [12]. In COPD and asthma, several types of inflammatory cells are increased [11]. Emphysema may result from the release of mediators and proteases that macrophages help to release, as well as the attraction of additional inflammatory cells (such as neutrophils) [11, 13].

2.1 Characteristics of COPD inflammation

There is a distinctive pattern of inflammation in COPD, marked by an increase of macrophages, T-lymphocytes, and B-lymphocytes as well as neutrophils in the airway lumen [13]. Both innate and adaptive immune responses are involved in the inflammatory response in COPD, and they are connected *via* the activation of dendritic cells. Smokers without airway restrictions also exhibit a similar pattern of inflammation and mediator expression, but in COPD, this inflammation is exacerbated and even increased during acute exacerbations brought on by bacterial or viral infection [13–15].

Smoke from cigarettes and other respiratory irritants can cause airway epithelial cells and surface macrophages to release a variety of chemotactic mediators, mainly chemokines, which draw circulation neutrophils, monocytes, and lymphocytes into the lungs [15]. Even after smoking is ceased, there is still inflammation, indicating that there are self-sustaining processes, but they have not yet been fully understood. Long-lived memory T-cells, bacterial colonization, or autoimmunity could be the source of the ongoing inflammation in COPD patients [13].

Increased neutrophil counts in the conducting airway lumen as well as in the airway walls are linked to the pathogenesis of COPD. The presence of increased macrophages in the parenchyma and small airways is closely correlated with the degree of emphysema [16]. CD8+ lymphocytes are present in peripheral smooth muscle, large and small airways, and the airway walls of emphysematous regions. Growth factors, cytokines, metalloproteinase, and serine proteinases are altered by inflammatory cell activation in COPD [17]. These modifications are thought to cause mucus hypersecretion, emphysematous modifications, damage to alveolar epithelial cells, and extracellular matrix degradation, particularly of lung elastin [13, 16].

Exacerbations of COPD are an intensification of the inflammatory response in the lungs. While bacterial infections, viral infections, or environmental toxins cause severe exacerbations, other causes of exacerbations are not known [18–20]. Increased lung inflammatory cell counts and inflammatory cell mediator release are the results of heightened inflammatory responses during COPD exacerbations, which enhances the pathological process linked to lung function loss [21]. During exacerbations, the number of neutrophils, lymphocytes, and eosinophils in the airways increases. Interleukin [IL]-8 and leukotriene-B4 are neutrophil chemoattractants, neutrophil degranulation products, C-reactive protein [CRP], eotaxin, and Regulated upon Activation, Normal T-cell Expressed, and Secreted [RANTES] are interleukin, and there are imbalances between proteinase and proteinase inhibitors [13, 18].

3. Doctor-patient communication

An important aspect of treating COPD is to educate patients and families about this chronic condition, its symptoms, and suggested pharmacological and nonpharmacological therapy. It is necessary to provide precise yet understandable explanations of the pathophysiology of COPD [22]. To comprehend patients' experiences and gauge the severity of the sickness, the clinician must be aware of common descriptions of air trapping, such as "air hunger," "unsatisfied" or "unrewarded" inhalation, "shallow breathing," "suffocating," and "cannot get a deep breath" [7, 23, 24].

High-quality care must include effective communication between patients and physicians, and patient-centered care models emphasize communication as a key enabler to reduce morbidity and death. The role of communication itself is unknown, although self-management programs for COPD patients include high-quality patient–clinician communication tactics that, in turn, result in better patient care and lower costs. Although better patient-clinician contact is frequently encouraged, it is unclear which health outcomes are aided by effective communication [25].

4. Prevention and early intervention

Lung function trajectories from birth or childhood to early adulthood have been documented in several birth-cohort studies. These trajectories may reflect the influence of potentially modifiable variables such as preterm delivery, smoke exposure, recurrent pulmonary infections, and persistent asthma during childhood. Interventions to enhance lung development and reduce the incidence of COPD in older age may concentrate on these aspects [26]. With the ultimate goal of identifying individuals with early disease who may benefit more from care, researchers are studying the early pathophysiologic alterations in COPD in light of this new understanding of lung function trajectories [27].

Epigenetic reprogramming of basal epithelial cells, which are crucial for efficient pulmonary host defense and epithelial remodeling following lung injury, is the first observable histologic change after exposure to cigarette smoke [28]. Distal airways show squamous metaplasia, ciliary failure, basal and goblet cell hyperplasia, and mucus hypersecretion because of epigenetic reprogramming of these cells. These changes result in a local inflammatory milieu that is vulnerable to injury and infection [29]. In fact, a gene expression examination of pulmonary epithelial samples from healthy smokers, healthy nonsmokers, and smokers with COPD showed that smokers, particularly those with COPD, reprogram the distal airways to more closely resemble proximal airways. This distal-to-proximal repatterning may be regulated by epidermal growth factor signaling in basal cells of tiny airways, which may be a potential therapeutic target [30, 31].

A number of pathogenic modifications in some persistent respiratory infections can be traced back to adaptive changes in the system that controls changes in epigenetic regulation of gene expression, which is a highly conserved evolutionary process [32]. Numerous preclinical investigations have focused heavily on the identification of epigenetic targets and the development of preventative measures against changes in epigenetic pathways [33].

DNA methylation of several genes has been reported in postmortem and lung biopsy samples from asthma patients [34]. Further research is required to determine the function of histone acetylation in asthma and to determine whether decreased histone deacetylase (HDAC) activity in asthma may result in higher expression of proinflammatory genes. The development of histone acetyltransferase (HAT) inhibitors that are therapeutically acceptable and efficient is still in the early stages and has to be further assessed [35, 36].

Similar mechanisms involving a combination of hypermethylation at some loci and hypomethylation at others have been identified in COPD patients [32]. Genes that are differentially expressed and controlled in COPD are connected to the PI3K/Akt and Nrf2 pathways. The phosphatase and tensin homolog (PTEN) and Nrf2 genes exhibit lower expression and activity as a result of hypermethylation in CpG islands [37]. PTEN is a regulator of PI3K/AKT signaling, which indirectly contributes to the inflammation and airway remodeling in COPD, while Nrf2 is implicated in anti-inflammatory. Epithelial dysfunction in cigarette smoke-mediated COPD has been linked to hypomethylation, which increases the expression of the HDAC6 promoter. There has been evidence of a decrease in the expression of HDACs 2, 3, 5, 8 and an increase in HDACs 4, 8 [35, 36].

The amount of water and mucin present in the fluids at the surface of the airways changes because of epithelial reprogramming brought on by prolonged exposure to cigarette smoke [38]. Through efficient mucus clearance, the normal structure and operation of this physiologic interface guard against airway blockage, irritation, and infection. Mucins, high-molecular-weight carbohydrate polymers made by goblet cells, have been linked to the clinical phenotype of chronic bronchitis and have been detected in higher amounts in the sputum of ever-smokers with COPD than in healthy controls [39]. Therefore, the concentration of airway mucin may both identify a possible treatment target and act as a diagnostic biomarker.

The polymeric Ig receptor (pIgR) in the healthy lung causes the small airway cells to produce dimeric immunoglobulin (Ig) A into the mucosal lumen. Secretory IgA (SIgA), still attached to the secretory component of pIgR, is released upon cleavage of pIgR at the luminal surface [40]. SIgA protects the respiratory epithelium from bacterial invasion. Smoking decreases the expression of pIgR, which results in a localized SIgA deficiency in the small airways [41]. Bacteria are able to enter respiratory epithelial cells in the absence of SIgA. Nuclear factor B is activated as a result, which causes and maintains airway inflammation [42]. Different lung microbial community architectures may help explain why some smokers do not acquire COPD, but it is still unclear whether specific microorganisms are responsible for the disease's progression and when it occurs [43].

According to these findings, airway remodeling, which may be a significant early pathologic lesion before the development of emphysema, may be caused by bacterial invasion. The small airways are, in fact, the main location of increased airway resistance among people with COPD, and these changes may take place even in the absence of other morphologic lung diseases, according to an additional study conducted in the late 1960s and early 1970s [44]. At first, it was thought that the small airways barely made a dent in the overall pulmonary resistance. Furthermore, it appears from histology and computed tomography (CT) studies that mild disease already exhibits distal airway constriction and dropout before overt emphysema manifests [45].

5. COPD risk factors

Understanding the symptoms of patients as well as the risk factors for COPD are crucial. In developed nations, 50 to 70% of people with COPD attributed their condition to cigarette smoking [7]. Additionally, genetics can increase your risk of getting COPD. The pathophysiology of COPD was linked to numerous genetic loci in a meta-analysis of genome-wide association studies [27, 46, 47]. The most often described genetic risk factor for COPD is serine protease 1-antitrypsin deficiency, which affects 1–3% of people with the disease [48]. Other risk factors for COPD include age, indoor and outdoor air pollution (including biomass fuels), and occupational exposure to dust, vapors, organic compounds, fumes, and chemicals, among others [7, 49].

6. Diagnosis

Dyspnea, a persistent cough, sputum production, and occasional wheezing are frequent symptoms of COPD. Unfortunately, delayed diagnosis is frequent, and many people remain undiagnosed until they have at least one exacerbation [50], which is frequently misdiagnosed as recurrent bronchitis [51]. To enhance patients' lung function, functional status, and QoL and to prevent exacerbations, early diagnosis and treatment are crucial [52]. If medical professionals include COPD in their differential diagnosis, it can be identified early [53]. For instance, COPD should be considered for patients over 40, even if they are nonsmokers when they have recurring acute bronchitis or severe colds that continue for weeks. It is noteworthy that women with COPD are more frequently undiagnosed than men with the same symptoms presumably because COPD has historically been viewed as a "male" disease [54]. Smoking is, however, one of several variables that have led to the increased incidence of COPD in women. By specifically focusing on respiratory symptoms (such as limitations in activity or lifestyle modifications brought on by shortness of breath), clinicians can also boost the likelihood of detecting COPD [55]. Patients frequently blame their "old, overweight, or out of shape" status for these symptoms [56]. To track changes in severity over time, helpful tools that are available to identify and evaluate baseline symptomatology might be used. The five statements that make up the modified Medical Research Council (mMRC) dyspnea scale describe a variety of dyspnea effects in descending order of severity [57]. The GOLD 2020 report recommends using this questionnaire. The substantial change in functional capacities from one grade to the next makes this questionnaire less suitable for monitoring patients over time [58], even though it may be beneficial for the initial detection of dyspnea and support evaluation for COPD [57, 58]. As an alternative, the COPD Assessment Test (CAT), which has eight items and scores them on a scale from 0 to 5, is helpful in determining how symptoms of COPD are affected [59]. A higher CAT score indicates poorer health. Thus, the CAT score more frequently manifests improvements brought on by medication, a slowing of the disease's progression, or exacerbations [60]. Prognostic models for COPD have recently made it possible to improve the criteria for choosing lung transplant patients [61]. The modified Medical Research Council dyspnea score (D), the 6-minute walk distance (E), the body mass index (B), the percent-predicted forced expiratory volume in 1 second (FEV1), the obstruction (O), and the body mass index (B) are all factors that the BODE index takes into account when estimating COPD survival [62].

When a patient reports having trouble breathing while exercising, the diagnosis usually starts with a clinical suspicion. Individuals with recurring respiratory issues (such as acute bronchitis, severe colds, chronic coughs, and excess sputum production), a history of risk factors, a reduction in activity due to dyspnea, and/or a family history of COPD are all considered symptomatic, at-risk individuals who need spirometry and evaluation for COPD [7, 63].

To confirm a COPD diagnosis, spirometry is crucial and required [64, 65]. It is helpful for tracking therapy effectiveness, maybe changing pharmaceutical dosages, and keeping track of illness development. The need for additional testing and referral to a lung specialist arises when rapid disease development is seen. The presence of a persistent or fixed airflow limitation is confirmed by a postbronchodilator FEV1 to forced vital capacity (FVC) ratio of less than 0.70 (10–15 minutes after 2–4 puffs of a short-acting bronchodilator) [66]. The maximum volume of air that can be forcedly exhaled after taking the deepest breath possible is known as FVC, and the maximum volume of air that can be forcedly expelled in the first second of an FVC maneuver is known as FEV1 [67].

Spirometry is not frequently utilized in clinical practice, despite guidelines [68]. Uncertainty regarding the value of a COPD diagnosis, a lack of time and resources, a lack of expertise with the procedure, and/or difficulties interpreting data are all reasons why spirometry is underutilized in primary care settings [7]. Spirometry, which may be carried out in primary care settings utilizing an office-based system and is a billable operation that is covered by payers, is nevertheless necessary to confirm a diagnosis of COPD [7, 69]. Spirometry may and should be performed in primary care offices because, although patients can be referred to specialists and hospitals for the test, follow-up may be limited [70].

Despite considerable disagreement over whether this is the optimum approach to quantify obstruction, the definition of COPD includes postbronchodilator spirometry demonstrating fixed airflow restriction defined as an FEV1/forced vital capacity (FVC) ratio of 0.70 [71, 72]. The GOLD Initiative has advocated using a set FEV1/FVC criterion to determine airflow obstruction [73]. The lower limit of normal (LLN), which is determined by age, race, sex, and height based on population-level data [74], is advised by the American Thoracic Society and the European Respiratory Society for FEV1/FVC [75–77]. Although the fixed cutoff is simpler to use, it may lead to more false positives in elderly patients who might then be given unnecessary treatment and to more false negatives in younger patients who might benefit from early intervention [77]. Currently, the most precise imaging method for emphysema diagnosis is computed tomography (CT) [78]. Extensive use of this technique, however, seems unwarranted due to the high cost and substantial radiation burden. Conversely, chest radiography is invariably performed in patients with COPD, but its accuracy in diagnosing emphysema is controversial [78–80]. When a diagnosis is made, a chest radiograph is typically taken, although repeat radiography is not advised in cases of stable disease. Lung function tests (LFT) determine the severity of COPD, and chest radiographs are primarily used to rule out comorbidities such as bronchogenic carcinoma, heart failure, and pneumonia [78, 79, 81].

7. Treatment

7.1 Pharmacology

According to GOLD recommendations, bronchodilators such as long-acting muscarinic antagonists (LAMA) are frequently used as the first line of treatment for the majority of symptomatic COPD patients [82, 83]. Acute worsening of coughing, shortness of breath, or mucus production beyond the normal day-to-day variance characterize COPD exacerbations [84, 85]. Exacerbations have a negative impact on the disease's natural history because they hasten the loss of lung function, raise mortality, deteriorate health, and increase cardiac events. The GOLD ABCD assessment method, which integrates exacerbation history as well as symptom burden to help guide pharmacologic care, shows that prevention of exacerbations is crucial in the management of COPD [86, 87]. Exacerbations in COPD patients can be considerably decreased with timely and suitable maintenance medication, particularly dual bronchodilators for maximal bronchodilation [87]. Pulmonary rehabilitation, follow-up appointments, aftercare, inhaler training, and patient education are further components of multidisciplinary disease management programs that help lower hospitalizations and readmissions for COPD patients [87, 88].

Little information was available to help clinicians decide whether to de-escalate from inhaled corticosteroids (ICS) in patients without frequent exacerbations who might not have as obvious a benefit. In the Study to Understand the Safety and Efficacy of ICS Withdrawal from Triple Therapy in COPD (SUNSET) trial, stable COPD patients were enrolled who were on long-term triple therapy and had experienced no more than one moderate or severe exacerbation in the previous year (FEV1 40–80% of expected) [89]. Patients with high baseline blood eosinophil levels (>300 cells/l) reported more exacerbations and a higher loss in lung function after ICS discontinuation [90]. A *post hoc* analysis of the Withdrawal of Inhaled Glucocorticoids and Exacerbations of COPD (WISDOM) trial discovered increased exacerbations after ICS withdrawal among participants with higher blood eosinophil counts at screening, further supporting the correlation between ICS use, exacerbation rate, and eosinophil count [91, 92]. Additionally, a secondary analysis of data from Informing the Pathway of COPD Treatment (IMPACT) modeled the eosinophil count as a continuous variable and revealed no difference in exacerbation reduction between the LAMA/LABA/ICS and LAMA/LABA arms at eosinophil counts below 100 cells/l but gradually greater treatment effects in the ICS-containing regimens with higher eosinophil levels [93–96]. The 2019 GOLD guidelines, which integrate serum eosinophil level, dyspnea, and exacerbation history to guide treatment escalation and de-escalation, incorporate these eosinophil findings. These study results highlight a shift in inhaler management toward a more precision-based approach [97].

Patients who frequently experience exacerbations despite receiving the maximum amount of inhaler therapy and those with eosinophil counts below 100 cells/l who are less likely to benefit from ICS are now frequently treated with oral medicines [98]. When administered as a preventative measure to COPD patients who are at a greater risk of exacerbation, azithromycin has been demonstrated to decrease exacerbations [99, 100]. Later studies supported its usage primarily for former smokers, as there was minimal evidence of a therapeutic benefit among active smokers [101]. QTc prolongation of the electrocardiogram and hearing loss are two known azithromycin adverse effects that need to be constantly evaluated in people taking the drug. Another potential issue is antibiotic resistance. The phosphodiesterase-4 inhibitor roflumilast is indicated for individuals with recurring exacerbations, FEV1 less than 50% expected, and chronic bronchitis phenotype [98].

7.2 Pulmonary rehabilitation

Pulmonary rehabilitation (PR) is an important strategy in the management of patients with stable COPD. Patients with COPD benefit from long-term rehabilitation, maintenance measures after rehabilitation, and the incorporation of education and strength training in PR [102]. Important elements of pulmonary rehabilitation include patient selection and assessment, psychosocial support, self-management education, dietary assistance, and exercise therapy, particularly inspiratory muscle training (IMT) [103]. Increased exercise tolerance, decreased anxiety and dyspnea, and improved self-efficacy and health-related quality of life are just some of the advantages associated with pulmonary rehabilitation [104, 105].

In order to restore the physical and mental health of individuals with chronic respiratory diseases, PR mixes aerobic exercise, muscle strength training, and education programs [100, 106]. PR has been demonstrated to improve health-related quality of life, boost functional ability, and lower hospitalizations. PR is still not used to its full potential despite its many advantages [107]. A lack of access and understanding among patients, payers, and clinicians is a likely cause. Greater learning opportunities and education regarding the process and benefits of pulmonary rehabilitation are required for general practitioners, nurse practitioners, and all other allied healthcare professionals [103, 108].

7.3 Lung volume reduction

Lung volume reduction (LVR) is an approach that removes the most damaged area of the lung so that healthier parts can work better. There are currently two procedures for LVR: LVR through surgery (LVRS) and LVR through the endobronchial valve (EBV) technique. It is one of the few surgical treatments for COPD patients [109].

Next to lung transplantation, LVRS continues to be one of the most valuable options for treatment for individuals with severe emphysema [110]. To achieve the best possible outcomes, careful patient selection in a multidisciplinary approach is essential. One of the important criteria for choosing patients is evaluating hyperinflation using body plethysmography [111]. For patients with severe emphysema, the goal of LVRS is to enhance lung function and quality of life by lowering dyspnea [110, 112]. It is important to help patients with severe emphysema enhance elastic recoil, decrease airflow restriction, and improve the mechanics of breathing by removing some of the most severely damaged lung tissue [110, 113].

Patients with both heterogeneous and homogeneous emphysema can benefit from LVRS since both conditions result in hyperinflation of the lung [114, 115]. However, the best evidence exists for heterogeneous upper-lobe predominant emphysema. The flattened diaphragm regains its dome-like shape by removing the parenchyma that is most affected and consequently reducing hyperinflation. This improves lung function and diaphragmatic muscle strength [110, 115].

EBV is a surgery where small, one-way valves are placed in the airways that supply the most emphysematous part of the lungs [112]. The valves allow air and mucus to exit when breathing out but prevent air from entering the target lobe of the lung when breathing in. As the target lobe contracts, the size of the lung also decreases, allowing for more efficient and comfortable breathing [110, 112, 116].

The major inclusion and exclusion criteria used to evaluate eligibility for surgery and/or bronchoscopic reduction are FEV1 and carbon monoxide diffusion capacity (DLCO) [110, 117]. According to the predetermined criteria from the NETT study, exercise ability varies by sex when it comes to surgical classification. High exercise capacity, as determined by the post-pulmonary rehab CPET, is defined as >25 W for women and > 40 W for men [110, 113].

Improved lung compliance is regarded as the primary benefit of LVR therapy because the lungs' size is better matched to the thorax in which they are located [118, 119]. As a result, there is an increase in lung elastic recoil at a constant thoracic inspiratory volume, an improvement in expiratory airflow, and a decrease in both dynamic and static hyperinflations. In fact, it is widely recognized that LVR therapy has an impact on FEV1, vital capacity (VC), total lung capacity (TLC), and residual volume (RV). The impact of LVR therapy on lung diffusing capacity and gas exchange, however, is far less well understood [110, 118, 119].

7.4 Targeted lung denervation and bronchial Rheoplasty

The pulmonary parasympathetic neural system, which regulates smooth muscle tone, reflex bronchoconstriction, mucus hypersecretion, and airway inflammation, is disrupted by targeted lung denervation (TLD) using bronchoscopic radiofrequency ablation [120, 121]. While a small randomized sham-controlled double-blind trial of TLD in patients with symptomatic moderate-to-severe COPD showed a decrease in respiratory adverse events, a larger randomized trial examining TLD's capacity to decrease COPD exacerbations is now enrolling participants [122]. Another bronchoscopic procedure is bronchial rheoplasty, which delivers nonthermal pulsed electric fields to the airways in order to ablate mucus-producing cells in patients with chronic bronchitis. Small, uncontrolled studies have indicated that this procedure reduces respiratory symptoms as well as goblet cell hyperplasia [123].

7.5 Lung transplantation

After all other forms of treatment have failed, lung transplantation (LTx) is a recognized alternative for individuals with end-stage lung illnesses. Patients may be eligible for lung transplantation if all other treatment options, such as oxygen therapy, noninvasive ventilation, lung volume reduction, and rehabilitation, have been used up or are not feasible [124].

LTx is a technique that can change a person's life, so both physicians and patients should take great care when choosing their COPD patients. The goal of patient selection is to increase survival due to the limited supply of organs. Not all COPD patients at the final stage qualify for LTx [125]. There are no randomized controlled trials that can be used to determine the advantages of LTx for COPD. The patient must weigh the risks and rewards in order to make a well-informed decision. The predicted survival probability of the underlying condition with LTx should be higher than that without LTx in order to improve a patient's prognosis and achieve a realistic survival benefit. Adults with end-stage chronic pulmonary illness who satisfy all of the following criteria should be given LTx consideration [126]:

- Poor waiting list survival and high risk of death (>50%) within 2 years if LTx is not performed;
- Good long-term prognosis following LTx; high likelihood (>80%) of 5-year posttransplant survival if appropriate graft function; poor waiting list survival.

When evaluating transplant candidates, it is essential to assess medical comorbidities, psychological issues, and the likelihood of rehabilitation. There are absolute and relative contraindications that need to be considered for patient selection to LTx. The absolute contraindications include [125–128]:

- Malignancy in the last 2 years
- With the exception of cutaneous squamous and basal cell tumors, a 5-year disease-free interval is desirable, especially in cases of malignant melanoma and

breast cancer, but at least 2-year disease-free survival is advised after definitive therapy for malignancy.

- Advanced organ dysfunction, albeit combined organ transplantation may be undertaken on an individual basis.
- Progressive systemic sclerosis, amyloidosis, and other systemic inflammatory disorders with primary lung involvement as well as widespread extrathoracic involvement
- Chronic extrapulmonary infection that cannot be treated and resolved.
- Lung transplantation has historically been viewed as being wholly contraindicated in cases of HIV infection and illness. This may become a relative contraindication, nevertheless, as the patient population gains more experience with the transplantation of other solid organs.
- Significant chest wall/spinal deformity.
- Medical noncompliance
- Uncontrolled psychiatric conditions that cannot be treated and resolved
- Lack of a stable social support system
- Substance abuse within the last 6 months, including smoking and alcohol abuse

Relative Contraindications include: [125, 126, 128, 129].

- Acute critical clinical conditions
- Age older than 65 years for single lung transplantation, 60 years for bilateral lung transplantation, and 55 years for heart-lung transplantation.
- Poor functional status without the potential for rehabilitation.
- Advanced malnutrition with a BMI less than 20 kg/m^2
- Obesity, with BMI greater than 30 kg/m^2
- Colonization or active infection with hard-to-treat or extremely pathogenic microorganisms
- Severe or symptomatic osteoporosis
- Comorbidities that have not yet resulted in advanced organ dysfunction
- Lack of adequate medical insurance coverage

Similar to other diseases, patients with COPD should be sent to a lung transplant clinic if their condition is progressing despite receiving the recommended amount of medical treatment and there are no evident contraindications [126]. A BODE (BMI, obstruction, dyspnea, and exercise capacity) score of 5 or higher with additional factors (frequent acute exacerbations, increase in BODE score of >1 over the past 24 months, pulmonary artery to aorta diameter of >1 on CT scan, and FEV1 25% predicted) present is recommended for LTx referral for a COPD patient. Despite receiving the most effective medical care, oxygen therapy, pulmonary rehabilitation, and, if necessary, nightly noninvasive positive pressure ventilation, clinical deterioration should be noted [126, 130, 131].

A COPD patient should be put on the waiting list for LTx if they have a BODE score of 7 to 10, as well as other conditions such as a FEV1 below 20% of expected and moderate-to-severe pulmonary hypertension [130]. People with end-stage COPD can undergo single- or double-lung transplants; however, people with α-1 AD may benefit more from a double-lung transplant [126, 132, 133].

7.6 Stem cell therapies

Anti-inflammatory drugs, corticosteroids, long-acting muscarinic antagonists, and 2-adrenoceptor agonists are some of the treatment options for COPD and asthma that are currently available. However, these medications cannot repair lung damage or significantly enhance patients' quality of life [134]. The molecular basis of COPD and asthma pathogeneses must therefore be better understood in order to create novel treatment and diagnostic strategies [134, 135].

Stem cells can differentiate into a variety of different lung cell types. Preclinical studies in animal models have suggested the regeneration of alveolar-like structures, repair of emphysematous lungs, and suppression of inflammatory responses. Regenerative therapies are currently divided into intrinsic cell therapy techniques and extrinsic therapeutic strategies [134, 136]. Extrinsic cell therapy involves injecting stem cells, such as embryonic stem cells (ESCs), induced pluripotent stem cells (iPSs), mesenchymal stem cells (MSCs), and human lung stem cells (hLSCs), through the trachea. Intrinsic therapy refers to the administration of tiny chemicals that can encourage the endogenous lung stem/progenitor cells to regenerate and replace damaged structures [135, 137].

According to a growing body of research, mesenchymal stem cells (MSCs) are excellent tools for cell-based therapy and regenerative medicine due to their multipotent differentiation self-renewal abilities and immunoregulatory capabilities, as well as their long-term *ex vivo* proliferation and paracrine effects [138, 139]. MSCs have been extensively investigated in relation to respiratory conditions like COPD, asthma, and idiopathic pulmonary fibrosis, and they are strong contenders for the healing of lung injury. Additionally, it has been established that the advantageous benefits of extracellular vehicles (EVs), in particular, of MSCs are primarily linked to their paracrine components [134]. Exosomes, microvesicles (MVs), microparticles (MPs), and their miRNA content have all been widely reported as potential therapeutic treatments for a variety of lung diseases [135, 140]. EVs also act as signaling molecules to mediate cell-cell communication, particularly between epithelial cells and the lung microenvironment. These vesicles have a higher safety profile and can be kept without losing function as compared to their mother MSCs. EVs have developed a reputation as advantageous substitutes for stem cell therapies because of their decreased immunogenicity and tumorigenicity and ease of management [134].

7.7 Gene therapy

Research and development in the field of gene therapy is expanding, and it may provide a durable cure for a number of difficult disorders, including chronic obstructive pulmonary disease (COPD). There are currently few curative treatments available for a number of respiratory disorders [141, 142]. The lung is an attractive organ for the delivery of targeted treatments, particularly for gene therapy, given its accessibility and the detection of genetic abnormalities in numerous respiratory disorders [143]. By introducing exogenous genetic material into cells or tissues to restore physiological protein expression and/or activity, gene therapy opens new therapeutic possibilities for the treatment of inherited and acquired disorders. The various preclinical research and clinical trials for the treatment of pulmonary arterial hypertension (PAH), idiopathic pulmonary fibrosis (IPF), cystic fibrosis (CF), asthma, COPD, alpha-1 antitrypsin (AAT) insufficiency, non-small cell lung cancer (NSCLC), and COVID-19 are excellent examples of the potential of gene therapy. Plasmid DNA, antisense oligonucleotides, mRNA, and peptide nucleic acids are examples of genetic materials. There are currently hundreds of clinical trials being conducted to investigate further options, and 23 gene therapy drugs have been approved for use in humans. The use of gene therapy in the treatment of respiratory disorders has gained momentum in recent years because of increased knowledge of the genetic and molecular causes of these conditions [144, 145].

Due to the complexity of the lung's anatomical and functional components and its particular collection of immune cells, local delivery approaches for gene therapy have had difficulty reaching the target [146]. With the ultimate goal of overcoming the physical and biological barriers imposed by the lung anatomy and innate immune defenses, multiple vectors have been developed and investigated to deliver cargoes for gene addition and gene-editing components.

Lung-targeted gene therapy has advanced over the past few years, with better vector design, improved transport, and increased efficacy. Asthma, CF, chronic obstructive pulmonary disease (COPD), lung cancer, PAH, IPF, AAT deficiency, and coronavirus disease 2019 (COVID-19) have all been the subject of additional research into the therapeutic potential of gene therapy [144, 147].

A number of intricate interactions between environmental variables and genetic problems lead to the complex disease known as COPD. Recent genetic evidence has reported several polymorphisms in protease (e.g., matrix metalloproteinase 1 and 2 (MMP1 and MMP12)), anti-protease (e.g., α1-antitrypsin, α1-antichymotrypsin, and α1-macroglobulin), antioxidant (e.g., heme oxygenase-1), cytokines (e.g., TGFβ1, TNF-α, IL-1 complex, IL-8, and IL-13), and other various genes (e.g., CFTR, human leukocyte antigen, vitamin D-binding protein, and β2 adrenergic receptor) that may be associated with COPD [147]. To assess the potential of genetic intervention for treating COPD, their implications and roles need to be further investigated. For instance, earlier research has shown that smoking is linked to lower CFTR levels and mucus clearance issues in COPD patients, indicating that CFTR gene transfer may be a potential therapeutic approach. The preclinical evaluation of gene transfer for treating COPD has been substantially hampered by the complex etiology of COPD and the lack of adequate animal models [144, 146].

7.7.1 Limitation of gene therapy

While no significant benefit was observed in clinical trials, earlier investigations using lung-targeted gene therapy demonstrated encouraging outcomes in animal models. Animal modeling itself, which falls short in faithfully simulating the precise aspects of human diseases, might be held accountable, at least in part, for the failure of successfully transferring preclinical findings to human investigations [145, 148]. Importantly, increasing evidence indicates that phenotypic and immunological variations between species may significantly reduce the efficiency of gene transfer in humans. When compared to human studies, gene therapy has produced contentious findings in experimental models of respiratory disorders in rodents [144]. This discrepancy may be at least partially explained by significant variations in lung cell biology between different species. Therapy outcomes are also influenced by additional patient selection characteristics, such as age and sex, as well as the severity of the disease at the time of therapy [144].

Many protective mechanisms work to preserve the integrity of the epithelial border because the lung epithelium is situated at the point where the human body and the environment being inhaled converge. The ability of gene vectors to reach the epithelium in sufficient concentrations may be restricted by this defense reaction, which may target inhaled foreign particles. Strong immune systems, both innate and acquired, may stop effective gene transfer [148]. It is important to note that the majority of lung disorders are accompanied by aberrant mucus production and inflammation, which may further lessen the effectiveness of gene transfer. It is true that the mucous layer that covers the epithelium retains and eliminates materials *via* the mucociliary clearance system, which may further lessen the efficiency of inhaled gene therapy [144]. In order to obtain long-lasting effects, repeated administration may be necessary, which presents the additional difficulty of anti-vector immunity. Further research on stem cells or progenitor cells may offer viable alternatives for future gene therapy trials, along with new recombinant vectors, to avoid recurrent administration.

7.7.2 Future perspectives

A growing body of research, which encourages more investigation into these techniques, is supporting the benefits of gene therapy for lung disorders [149]. To increase the success rate, it is essential to recognize the constraints and create tools and strategies to go beyond the obstacles that are encountered. The development of disease models that are of high fidelity and are species-specific, as well as novel and improved vectors that can avoid degradation and bypass the immune response after delivery, will contribute to advancements in the field of gene therapy for respiratory diseases [150]. A further benefit that can be taken advantage of in the design of gene transfer approaches for the lung is the simplicity of access to the airways and respiratory epithelial surface through noninvasive (intranasal aerosolization) or minimally invasive (intratracheal aerosolization or bronchoscopy) procedures. All of these elements should work together to increase transduction and transfection rates, facilitate effective expression with minimal off-target consequences, and enhance long-term safety [150, 151].

8. Conclusion

COPD is a global health concern with a high prevalence and significant morbidity and mortality rates. It is characterized by persistent respiratory symptoms and airflow limitation due to exposure to noxious particles or gases. The primary risk factor in

DOI: http://dx.doi.org/10.5772/intechopen.1003820

high-income nations is smoking, while in low-income countries, indoor cooking and occupational exposure play a significant role. COPD is a complex disease with varied clinical manifestations, but it is commonly classified and staged based on lung function, symptoms, and exacerbation history.

The GOLD recommendations emphasize the use of LAMAs as the first line of treatment for symptomatic COPD patients. COPD exacerbations, characterized by acute worsening of respiratory symptoms, significantly increase the disease's rate of progression and worsen patient outcomes. The GOLD ABCD assessment method, which considers both exacerbation history and symptom burden, highlights the importance of preventing exacerbations in COPD management. TLD using bronchoscopic radiofrequency ablation has shown promise in disrupting the pulmonary parasympathetic neural system, which plays a role in regulating various aspects of COPD pathophysiology. The procedure may reduce respiratory adverse events in patients with symptomatic moderate-to-severe COPD. However, larger randomized trials are currently underway to provide more definitive evidence regarding its clinical effectiveness.

Stem cells as potential therapeutic tools can differentiate into several different lung cell types such as the alveolar epithelial cells. Due to their therapeutic capabilities, including anti-inflammatory and immunoregulatory properties, regeneration ability, as well as many other advantageous features, MSCs have recently acquired prominence in the treatment of many respiratory disorders. They are effective agents for cell-based therapy and regenerative medicine because of their multipotent differentiation, self-renewal capacities, and paracrine effects. The effective management and treatment of asthma, COPD, and several other diseases with inflammatory pathophysiology has future potential when epigenetics and gene-silencing technologies are combined with improved delivery techniques and biosafety. The field of gene therapy for respiratory diseases is growing and has vast potential. The development of genetic testing has shown altered gene expression profiles in a number of respiratory diseases.

Conflict of interest

The authors declare that they have no competing interest.

Author details

Biruk Getahun[1*], Abebe Ayalew Bekel[2], Dessalegn Demeke Ayalew[1], Melkamu Demewez Gebeye[3], Dagnachew Zemene[4] and Erstu Legese Beyene[5]

1 Department of Medical Physiology, School of Medicine, College of Medicine and Health Sciences, Bahir Dar University, Bahir Dar, Ethiopia

2 Department of Human Anatomy, School of Medicine, College of Medicine and Health Sciences, Bahir Dar University, Bahir Dar, Ethiopia

3 Faculty of Civil and Water Resource Engineering, Department of Structural Engineering, Bahir Dar Institute of Technology, Bahir Dar University, Ethiopia

4 Department of Plastic Surgery, School of Medicine, Yekatit 12 Hospital Medical College, Addis Ababa, Ethiopia

5 Department of Political Science and International Relations, College of Social Sciences and Humanities, Injebara University, Injebara, Ethiopia

*Address all correspondence to: birukkgetahun@gmail.com

DOI: http://dx.doi.org/10.5772/intechopen.1003820

References

[1] Ferrera MC, Labaki WW, Han MK. Advances in chronic obstructive pulmonary disease. Annual Review of Medicine. 2021;**72**:119-134

[2] Chen S, Kuhn M, Prettner K, Yu F, Yang T, Bärnighausen T, et al. The global economic burden of chronic obstructive pulmonary disease for 204 countries and territories in 2020-50: A health-augmented macroeconomic modelling study. The Lancet Global Health. 2023;**11**(8):e1183-e1e93

[3] Agustí A, Celli BR, Criner GJ, Halpin D, Anzueto A, Barnes P, et al. Global initiative for chronic obstructive lung disease 2023 report: GOLD executive summary. American Journal of Respiratory and Critical Care Medicine. 2023;**207**(7):819-837

[4] Brandsma CA, Van den Berge M, Hackett TL, Brusselle G, Timens W. Recent advances in chronic obstructive pulmonary disease pathogenesis: From disease mechanisms to precision medicine. The Journal of Pathology. 2020;**250**(5):624-635

[5] Postma DS, Kerkhof M, Boezen HM, Koppelman GH. Asthma and chronic obstructive pulmonary disease: Common genes, common environments? American Journal of Respiratory and Critical Care Medicine. 2011;**183**(12):1588-1594

[6] Hogg JC, Timens W. The pathology of chronic obstructive pulmonary disease. Annual Review of Pathology: Mechanisms of Disease. 2009;**4**:435-459

[7] Yawn BP, Mintz ML, Doherty DE. GOLD in practice: Chronic obstructive pulmonary disease treatment and management in the primary care setting. International Journal of Chronic Obstructive Pulmonary Disease. 2021;**16**:289-299

[8] Roca M, Verduri A, Corbetta L, Clini E, Fabbri LM, Beghé B. Mechanisms of acute exacerbation of respiratory symptoms in chronic obstructive pulmonary disease. European Journal of Clinical Investigation. 2013;**43**(5):510-521

[9] Shin K-C. Physical activity in chronic obstructive pulmonary disease: Clinical impact and risk factors. The Korean Journal of Internal Medicine. 2018;**33**(1):75

[10] Jones PW, Watz H, Wouters EF, Cazzola M. COPD: The patient perspective. International Journal of Chronic Obstructive Pulmonary Disease. 2016;**11**(Suppl. 1):13-20

[11] Baraldo S, Turato G, Saetta M. Pathophysiology of the small airways in chronic obstructive pulmonary disease. Respiration. 2012;**84**(2):89-97

[12] Mortezaee K, Majidpoor J. CD8+ T cells in SARS-CoV-2 induced disease and cancer—Clinical perspectives. Frontiers in Immunology. 2022;**13**:864298

[13] Barnes PJ. Inflammatory mechanisms in patients with chronic obstructive pulmonary disease. Journal of Allergy and Clinical Immunology. 2016;**138**(1):16-27

[14] Oudijk ED, Lammers JJ, Koenderman L. Systemic inflammation in chronic obstructive pulmonary disease. European Respiratory Journal. 2003;**22**(46 Suppl.):5s-13s

[15] Rovina N, Koutsoukou A, Koulouris NG. Inflammation and immune

response in COPD: Where do we stand? Mediators of Inflammation. 2013;**2013**

[16] Barnes PJ. The cytokine network in chronic obstructive pulmonary disease. American Journal of Respiratory Cell and Molecular Biology. 2009;**41**(6):631-638

[17] Eyraud E, Maurat E, Sac-Epée J-M, Henrot P, Zysman M, Esteves P, et al. Short-range interactions between fibrocytes and CD8+ T cells in COPD bronchial inflammatory response. eLife. 2023;**12**:RP85875

[18] Sethi S, Mahler DA, Marcus P, Owen CA, Yawn B, Rennard S. Inflammation in COPD: Implications for management. The American Journal of Medicine. 2012;**125**(12):1162-1170

[19] Gayle AV, Quint JK, Fuertes EI. Understanding the relationships between environmental factors and exacerbations of COPD. Expert Review of Respiratory Medicine. 2021;**15**(1):39-50

[20] Rabe KF, Hurd S, Anzueto A, Barnes PJ, Buist SA, Calverley P, et al. Global strategy for the diagnosis, management, and prevention of chronic obstructive pulmonary disease: GOLD executive summary. American Journal of Respiratory and Critical Care Medicine. 2007;**176**(6):532-555

[21] Crisan L, Wong N, Sin DD, Lee HM. Karma of cardiovascular disease risk factors for prevention and management of major cardiovascular events in the context of acute exacerbations of chronic obstructive pulmonary disease. Frontiers in Cardiovascular Medicine. 2019;**6**:79

[22] Hurst JR, Winders T, Worth H, Bhutani M, Gruffydd-Jones K, Stolz D, et al. A patient charter for chronic obstructive pulmonary disease. Advances in Therapy. 2021;**38**:11-23

[23] O'Donnell DE, Webb KA, Neder JA. Lung hyperinflation in COPD: Applying physiology to clinical practice. COPD Research and Practice. 2015;**1**(1):1-12

[24] Langer D, Ciavaglia CE, Neder JA, Webb KA, O'Donnell DE. Lung hyperinflation in chronic obstructive pulmonary disease: Mechanisms, clinical implications and treatment. Expert Review of Respiratory Medicine. 2014;**8**(6):731-749

[25] Slatore CG, Cecere LM, Reinke LF, Ganzini L, Udris EM, Moss BR, et al. Patient-clinician communication: Associations with important health outcomes among veterans with COPD. Chest. 2010;**138**(3):628-634

[26] Ambrosino N, Bertella E. Lifestyle interventions in prevention and comprehensive management of COPD. Breathe. 2018;**14**(3):186-194

[27] Celli BR, Singh D, Vogelmeier C, Agusti A. New perspectives on chronic obstructive pulmonary disease. International Journal of Chronic Obstructive Pulmonary Disease. 2022;**17**:2127-2136

[28] Komlósi ZI, van de Veen W, Kovács N, Szűcs G, Sokolowska M, O'Mahony L, et al. Cellular and molecular mechanisms of allergic asthma. Molecular Aspects of Medicine. 2022;**85**:100995

[29] Hewitt RJ, Lloyd CM. Regulation of immune responses by the airway epithelial cell landscape. Nature Reviews Immunology. 2021;**21**(6):347-362

[30] Blackburn JB, Li NF, Bartlett NW, Richmond BW. An update in club cell biology and its potential relevance to chronic obstructive pulmonary disease. American Journal of Physiology-Lung Cellular and Molecular Physiology. 2023;**324**(5):L652-LL65

[31] Bartel S, Bhakta N, Christenson S. More than meets the eye: Cigarette smoke induces genomic changes in the small airway epithelium independent of histologic changes. American Journal of Respiratory and Critical Care Medicine. 1 Aug 2017;**196**(3):260-262

[32] Schamberger AC, Mise N, Meiners S, Eickelberg O. Epigenetic mechanisms in COPD: Implications for pathogenesis and drug discovery. Expert Opinion on Drug Discovery. 2014;**9**(6):609-628

[33] Kabesch M, Adcock IM. Epigenetics in asthma and COPD. Biochimie. 2012;**94**(11):2231-2241

[34] Al TA. Role of DNA Methylation in Common Disease: Analysis of Two Asthma-Associated Regions. Montreal: McGill University (Canada); 2018

[35] Afzal S, Ramzan K, Waqar AB. Alternative approaches for the treatment of asthma and COPD: Focus on cell-based therapies, epigenetics, and gene silencing approaches. Advancements in Life Sciences. 2020;**7**(3):181-189

[36] Niederberger E, Resch E, Parnham MJ, Geisslinger G. Drugging the pain epigenome. Nature Reviews Neurology. 2017;**13**(7):434-447

[37] Chen Y-C, Tsai Y-H, Wang C-C, Liu S-F, Chen T-W, Fang W-F, et al. Epigenome-wide association study on asthma and chronic obstructive pulmonary disease overlap reveals aberrant DNA methylations related to clinical phenotypes. Scientific Reports. 2021;**11**(1):5022

[38] Hill DB, Button B, Rubinstein M, Boucher RC. Physiology and pathophysiology of human airway mucus. Physiological Reviews. 2022;**102**(4):1757-1836

[39] Ghio AJ, Pavlisko EN, Roggli VL, Todd NW, Sangani RG. Cigarette smoke particle-induced lung injury and iron homeostasis. International Journal of Chronic Obstructive Pulmonary Disease. 2022;**17**:117-140

[40] de Fays C, Carlier FM, Gohy S, Pilette C. Secretory immunoglobulin a immunity in chronic obstructive respiratory diseases. Cell. 2022;**11**(8):1324

[41] Polosukhin VV, Richmond BW, Du R-H, Cates JM, Wu P, Nian H, et al. Secretory IgA deficiency in individual small airways is associated with persistent inflammation and remodeling. American Journal of Respiratory and Critical Care Medicine. 2017;**195**(8):1010-1021

[42] Gasaly N, Hermoso MA, Gotteland M. Butyrate and the fine-tuning of colonic homeostasis: Implication for inflammatory bowel diseases. International Journal of Molecular Sciences. 2021;**22**(6):3061

[43] Natalini JG, Singh S, Segal LN. The dynamic lung microbiome in health and disease. Nature Reviews Microbiology. 2023;**21**(4):222-235

[44] Hogg JC, Paré PD, Hackett T-L. The contribution of small airway obstruction to the pathogenesis of chronic obstructive pulmonary disease. Physiological Reviews. 2017;**97**(2):529-552

[45] Lynch DA, Austin JH, Hogg JC, Grenier PA, Kauczor H-U, Bankier AA, et al. CT-definable subtypes of chronic obstructive pulmonary disease: A statement of the Fleischner society. Radiology. 2015;**277**(1):192-205

[46] Shrine N, Izquierdo AG, Chen J, Packer R, Hall RJ, Guyatt AL,

et al. Multi-ancestry genome-wide association analyses improve resolution of genes and pathways influencing lung function and chronic obstructive pulmonary disease risk. Nature Genetics. 2023;**55**(3):410-422

[47] Cho MH, McDonald M-LN, Zhou X, Mattheisen M, Castaldi PJ, Hersh CP, et al. Risk loci for chronic obstructive pulmonary disease: A genome-wide association study and meta-analysis. The Lancet Respiratory Medicine. 2014;**2**(3):214-225

[48] Köhnlein T, Welte T. Alpha-1 antitrypsin deficiency: Pathogenesis, clinical presentation, diagnosis, and treatment. The American Journal of Medicine. 2008;**121**(1):3-9

[49] Kc R, Shukla SD, Gautam SS, Hansbro PM, O'Toole RF. The role of environmental exposure to non-cigarette smoke in lung disease. Clinical and Translational Medicine. 2018;**7**(1):1-12

[50] Mincheva R, Ekerljung L, Bjerg A, Axelsson M, Popov TA, Lundbäck B, et al. Frequent cough in unsatisfactory controlled asthma–results from the population-based West Sweden asthma study. Respiratory Research. 2014;**15**:1-11

[51] Stephens MB, Yew KS. Diagnosis of chronic obstructive pulmonary disease. American Family Physician. 2008;**78**(1):87-92

[52] Sandelowsky H, Weinreich UM, Aarli BB, Sundh J, Høines K, Stratelis G, et al. COPD–do the right thing. BMC Family Practice. 2021;**22**(1):1-17

[53] Ko FW, Chan KP, Hui DS, Goddard JR, Shaw JG, Reid DW, et al. Acute exacerbation of COPD. Respirology. 2016;**21**(7):1152-1165

[54] Bouza E, Alvar A, Almagro P, Alonso T, Ancochea J, Barbe F, et al. Chronic obstructive pulmonary disease (COPD) in Spain and the different aspects of its social impact: A multidisciplinary opinion document. Revista Española de Quimioterapia. 2020;**33**(1):49

[55] Vogelmeier CF, Roman-Rodriguez M, Singh D, Han MK, Rodriguez-Roisin R, Ferguson GT. Goals of COPD treatment: Focus on symptoms and exacerbations. Respiratory Medicine. 2020;**166**:105938

[56] Buttery SC, Zysman M, Vikjord SA, Hopkinson NS, Jenkins C, Vanfleteren LE. Contemporary perspectives in COPD: Patient burden, the role of gender and trajectories of multimorbidity. Respirology. 2021;**26**(5):419-441

[57] Yorke J, Khan N, Garrow A, Tyson S, Singh D, Vestbo J, et al. Evaluation of the individual activity descriptors of the mMRC breathlessness scale: A mixed method study. International Journal of Chronic Obstructive Pulmonary Disease. 2022;**17**:2289-2299

[58] Grønseth R, Vollmer WM, Hardie JA, Ólafsdóttir IS, Lamprecht B, Buist AS, et al. Predictors of dyspnoea prevalence: Results from the BOLD study. European Respiratory Journal. 2014;**43**(6):1610-1620

[59] Martinez CH, Murray S, Barr RG, Bleecker E, Bowler RP, Christenson SA, et al. Respiratory symptoms items from the COPD assessment test identify ever-smokers with preserved lung function at higher risk for poor respiratory outcomes. An analysis of the subpopulations and intermediate outcome measures in COPD study cohort. Annals of the American Thoracic Society. 2017;**14**(5):636-642

[60] Wageck B, Cox NS, Holland AE. Recovery following acute exacerbations

of chronic obstructive pulmonary disease–A review. COPD: Journal of Chronic Obstructive Pulmonary Disease. 2019;**16**(1):93-103

[61] Sharma K, Jain A, Takhar R, Sudan D, Goyal V, Goel N, et al. Prognostic assessment in COPD patients: BODE index and the health-related quality of life. The Journal of Association of Chest Physicians. 2020;**8**(1):6

[62] Vieira EB, Degani-Costa LH, Amorim BC, Oliveira LB, Miranda-Silva T, Sperandio PC, et al. Modified BODE index to predict mortality in individuals with COPD: The role of 4-min step test. Respiratory Care. 2020;**65**(7):977-983

[63] MacLeod M, Papi A, Contoli M, Beghé B, Celli BR, Wedzicha JA, et al. Chronic obstructive pulmonary disease exacerbation fundamentals: Diagnosis, treatment, prevention and disease impact. Respirology. 2021;**26**(6):532-551

[64] Soriano JB, Zielinski J, Price D. Screening for and early detection of chronic obstructive pulmonary disease. The Lancet. 2009;**374**(9691):721-732

[65] Buffels J, Degryse J, Heyrman J, Decramer M. Office spirometry significantly improves early detection of COPD in general practice: The DIDASCO study. Chest. 2004;**125**(4):1394-1399

[66] McKleroy W, Shing T, Anderson WH, Arjomandi M, Awan HA, Barjaktarevic I, et al. Longitudinal follow-up of participants with tobacco exposure and preserved spirometry. Journal of the American Medical Association. 2023;**330**(5):442-453

[67] Sharan RV, Abeyratne UR, Swarnkar VR, Claxton S, Hukins C, Porter P. Predicting spirometry readings using cough sound features and regression. Physiological Measurement. 2018;**39**(9):095001

[68] Han MK, Kim MG, Mardon R, Renner P, Sullivan S, Diette GB, et al. Spirometry utilization for COPD: How do we measure up? Chest. 2007;**132**(2):403-409

[69] Nolte E, Knai C, Organization WH. Assessing Chronic Disease Management in European Health Systems: Country Reports: World Health Organization. United Kingdom: Regional Office for Europe; 2015

[70] Yu WC, Fu SN, Tai EL-B, Yeung YC, Kwong KC, Chang Y, et al. Spirometry is underused in the diagnosis and monitoring of patients with chronic obstructive pulmonary disease (COPD). International Journal of Chronic Obstructive Pulmonary Disease. 2013;**8**:389-395

[71] Meijer CA, Kokje VB, van Tongeren RB, Hamming JF, van Bockel JH, Möller GM, et al. An association between chronic obstructive pulmonary disease and abdominal aortic aneurysm beyond smoking: Results from a case–control study. European Journal of Vascular and Endovascular Surgery. 2012;**44**(2):153-157

[72] Chhabra S. Interpretation of spirometry: Selection of predicted values and defining abnormality. The Indian Journal of Chest Diseases & Allied Sciences. 2015;**57**(2):91-105

[73] Hansen JE, Sun X-G, Wasserman K. Spirometric criteria for airway obstruction: Use percentage of FEV1/FVC ratio below the fifth percentile, not< 70%. Chest. 2007;**131**(2):349-355

[74] McDonnell MJ, Harrison M, Rutherford RM. Is the GOLD guideline

for diagnosing obstruction in COPD discriminatory in predicting severe future COPD-related exacerbations and death? Breathe. 2021;**17**(4)

[75] Kainu A, Timonen K, Lindqvist A, Piirilä P. GOLD criteria overestimate airflow limitation in one-third of cases in the general Finnish population. ERJ Open Research. 2016;**2**(4)

[76] Qaseem A, Wilt TJ, Weinberger SE, Hanania NA, Criner G, van der Molen T, et al. Diagnosis and management of stable chronic obstructive pulmonary disease: A clinical practice guideline update from the American College of Physicians, American College of Chest Physicians, American Thoracic Society, and European Respiratory Society. Annals of Internal Medicine. 2011;**155**(3):179-191

[77] Hankinson JL, Kawut SM, Shahar E, Smith LJ, Stukovsky KH, Barr RG. Performance of American Thoracic Society-recommended spirometry reference values in a multiethnic sample of adults: The multi-ethnic study of atherosclerosis (MESA) lung study. Chest. 2010;**137**(1):138-145

[78] Miniati M, Monti S, Stolk J, Mirarchi G, Falaschi F, Rabinovich R, et al. Value of chest radiography in phenotyping chronic obstructive pulmonary disease. European Respiratory Journal. 2008;**31**(3):509-515

[79] Shaker SB, Dirksen A, Bach KS, Mortensen J. Imaging in chronic obstructive pulmonary disease. COPD: Journal of Chronic Obstructive Pulmonary Disease. 2007;**4**(2):143-161

[80] Coppini G, Miniati M, Monti S, Paterni M, Favilla R, Ferdeghini EM. A computer-aided diagnosis approach for emphysema recognition in chest radiography. Medical Engineering & Physics. 2013;**35**(1):63-73

[81] Urban T, Gassert FT, Frank M, Willer K, Noichl W, Buchberger P, et al. Qualitative and quantitative assessment of emphysema using dark-field chest radiography. Radiology. 2022;**303**(1):119-127

[82] Hurst JR, Dilleen M, Morris K, Hills S, Emir B, Jones R. Factors influencing treatment escalation from long-acting muscarinic antagonist monotherapy to triple therapy in patients with COPD: A retrospective THIN-database analysis. International Journal of Chronic Obstructive Pulmonary Disease. 2018;**13**:781-792

[83] Fukuda N, Horita N, Kaneko A, Goto A, Kaneko T, Ota E, et al. Long-acting muscarinic antagonist (LAMA) plus long-acting beta-agonist (LABA) versus LABA plus inhaled corticosteroid (ICS) for stable chronic obstructive pulmonary disease. Cochrane Database of Systematic Reviews. 2023;**6**

[84] Celli BR, Fabbri LM, Aaron SD, Agusti A, Brook R, Criner GJ, et al. An updated definition and severity classification of chronic obstructive pulmonary disease exacerbations: The Rome proposal. American Journal of Respiratory and Critical Care Medicine. 2021;**204**(11):1251-1258

[85] Hughes R, Rapsomaniki E, Janson C, Keen C, Make BJ, Burgel P-R, et al. Frequent productive cough: Symptom burden and future exacerbation risk among patients with asthma and/or COPD in the NOVELTY study. Respiratory Medicine. 2022;**200**:106921

[86] Singh D, Agusti A, Anzueto A, Barnes PJ, Bourbeau J, Celli BR, et al. Global strategy for the diagnosis, management, and prevention of chronic obstructive lung disease: The GOLD science committee report 2019. European Respiratory Journal. 2019;**53**(5):1900164

[87] Bollmeier SG, Hartmann AP. Management of chronic obstructive pulmonary disease: A review focusing on exacerbations. American Journal of Health-System Pharmacy. 2020;**77**(4):259-268

[88] Vogelmeier CF, Criner GJ, Martinez FJ, Anzueto A, Barnes PJ, Bourbeau J, et al. Global strategy for the diagnosis, management, and prevention of chronic obstructive lung disease 2017 report. GOLD executive summary. American Journal of Respiratory and Critical Care Medicine. 2017;**195**(5):557-582

[89] Chapman KR, Hurst JR, Frent S-M, Larbig M, Fogel R, Guerin T, et al. Long-term triple therapy de-escalation to indacaterol/glycopyrronium in patients with chronic obstructive pulmonary disease (SUNSET): A randomized, double-blind, triple-dummy clinical trial. American Journal of Respiratory and Critical Care Medicine. 2018;**198**(3):329-339

[90] Yun JH, Lamb A, Chase R, Singh D, Parker MM, Saferali A, et al. Blood eosinophil count thresholds and exacerbations in patients with chronic obstructive pulmonary disease. Journal of Allergy and Clinical Immunology. 2018;**141**(6):2037-2047 e10

[91] Watz H, Tetzlaff K, Wouters EF, Kirsten A, Magnussen H, Rodriguez-Roisin R, et al. Blood eosinophil count and exacerbations in severe chronic obstructive pulmonary disease after withdrawal of inhaled corticosteroids: A post-hoc analysis of the WISDOM trial. The Lancet Respiratory Medicine. 2016;**4**(5):390-398

[92] Harries TH, Rowland V, Corrigan CJ, Marshall IJ, McDonnell L, Prasad V, et al. Blood eosinophil count, a marker of inhaled corticosteroid effectiveness in preventing COPD exacerbations in post-hoc RCT and observational studies: Systematic review and meta-analysis. Respiratory Research. 2020;**21**(1):1-15

[93] Koarai A, Yamada M, Ichikawa T, Fujino N, Kawayama T, Sugiura H. Triple versus LAMA/LABA combination therapy for patients with COPD: A systematic review and meta-analysis. Respiratory Research. 2021;**22**(1):1-11

[94] Kocks J, Ferreira AJ, Bakke P, van Schayck OC, Ekroos H, Tzanakis N, et al. Investigating the rationale for COPD maintenance therapy prescription across Europe, findings from a multi-country study. NPJ Primary Care Respiratory Medicine. 2023;**33**(1):18

[95] Fuschillo S, Molino A, Stellato C, Motta A, Maniscalco M. Blood eosinophils as biomarkers of therapeutic response to chronic obstructive pulmonary disease: Still work in progress. European Journal of Internal Medicine. 2019;**68**:1-5

[96] Suissa S, Dell'Aniello S, Ernst P. Triple inhaler versus dual bronchodilator therapy in COPD: Real-world effectiveness on mortality. COPD: Journal of Chronic Obstructive Pulmonary Disease. 2022;**19**(1):1-9

[97] Kerkhof M, Tran TN, van den Berge M, Brusselle GG, Gopalan G, Jones RC, et al. Association between blood eosinophil count and risk of readmission for patients with asthma: Historical cohort study. PLoS One. 2018;**13**(7):e0201143

[98] Rhee CK, Kim DK. Role of phosphodiesterase-4 inhibitors in chronic obstructive pulmonary disease. The Korean Journal of Internal Medicine. 2020;**35**(2):276

[99] Albert RK, Connett J, Bailey WC, Casaburi R, Cooper JAD Jr, Criner GJ,

et al. Azithromycin for prevention of exacerbations of COPD. New England Journal of Medicine. 2011;**365**(8):689-698

[100] Holland AE, Wadell K, Spruit MA. How to adapt the pulmonary rehabilitation programme to patients with chronic respiratory disease other than COPD. European Respiratory Review. 2013;**22**(130):577-586

[101] Naderi N, Assayag D, Kaddaha Z, Joubert A, Ouellet I, Drouin I, et al. Long-term azithromycin therapy to reduce acute exacerbations in patients with severe chronic obstructive pulmonary disease. Respiratory Medicine. 2018;**138**:129-136

[102] Ma H, Dai M, Wu S, Zhao Z, Zhang Y, Zhao F, et al. Pulmonary rehabilitation ameliorates regional lung function in chronic obstructive pulmonary disease: A prospective single-arm clinical trial. Annals of Translational Medicine. 2022;**10**(16):891

[103] Getahun B, Bekel AA. Current and Contemporary Developments in Pulmonary Rehabilitation. Chronic Obstructive Pulmonary Disease-A Compendium of Medicine and the Humanities. IntechOpen; 14 Nov 2022

[104] Spruit MA, Vanderhoven-Augustin I, Janssen PP, Wouters EF. Integration of pulmonary rehabilitation in COPD. The Lancet. 2008;**371**(9606):12-13

[105] Zeng Y, Jiang F, Chen Y, Chen P, Cai S. Exercise assessments and trainings of pulmonary rehabilitation in COPD: A literature review. International Journal of Chronic Obstructive Pulmonary Disease. 2018;**13**:2013-2023

[106] Osadnik CR, Singh S. Pulmonary rehabilitation for obstructive lung disease. Respirology. 2019;**24**(9):871-878

[107] Arnold MT, Dolezal BA, Cooper CB. Pulmonary rehabilitation for chronic obstructive pulmonary disease: Highly effective but often overlooked. Tuberculosis and Respiratory Diseases. 2020;**83**(4):257

[108] McCarthy B, Casey D, Devane D, Murphy K, Murphy E, Lacasse Y. Pulmonary rehabilitation for chronic obstructive pulmonary disease. Cochrane Database of Systematic Reviews. 2015;(2)

[109] Marchetti N, Criner GJ, editors. Surgical approaches to treating emphysema: Lung volume reduction surgery, bullectomy, and lung transplantation. In: Seminars in Respiratory and Critical Care Medicine. Thieme Medical Publishers; 2015

[110] Gordon M, Duffy S, Criner GJ. Lung volume reduction surgery or bronchoscopic lung volume reduction: Is there an algorithm for allocation? Journal of Thoracic Disease. 2018;**10**(Suppl. 23):S2816

[111] D'Ascanio M, Viccaro F, Calabrò N, Guerrieri G, Salvucci C, Pizzirusso D, et al. Assessing static lung hyperinflation by whole-body plethysmography, helium dilution, and impulse oscillometry system (IOS) in patients with COPD. International Journal of Chronic Obstructive Pulmonary Disease. 2020;**15**:2583-2589

[112] England N. Clinical Commissioning Policy Proposition: Lung volume Reduction by Surgery or Endobronchial Valve for Severe Emphysema in Adults. Jan 2022;(1622):200806P

[113] Minervini F, Kestenholz PB, Paolini V, Pesci A, Libretti L, Bertolaccini L, et al. Surgical and endoscopic treatment for COPD: Patients selection, techniques and results. Journal

of Thoracic Disease. 2018;**10**(Suppl. 27):S3344

[114] Valipour A, Slebos D-J, Herth F, Darwiche K, Wagner M, Ficker JH, et al. Endobronchial valve therapy in patients with homogeneous emphysema. Results from the IMPACT study. American Journal of Respiratory and Critical Care Medicine. 2016;**194**(9):1073-1082

[115] van Dijk M, Klooster K, Ten Hacken NH, Sciurba F, Kerstjens HA, Slebos D-J. The effects of lung volume reduction treatment on diffusing capacity and gas exchange. European Respiratory Review. 2020;**29**(158):190171

[116] Cooper J, Trulock E, Triantafillou A, Patterson G, Pohl M, Deloney P, et al. Bilateral pneumectomy (volume reduction) for chronic obstructive pulmonary disease. The Journal of Thoracic and Cardiovascular Surgery. 1995;**109**(1):106-119

[117] Cerfolio RJ, Bryant AS. Different diffusing capacity of the lung for carbon monoxide as predictors of respiratory morbidity. The Annals of Thoracic Surgery. 2009;**88**(2):405-411

[118] Fessler HE, Scharf SM, Ingenito EP, McKenna RJ Jr, Sharafkhaneh A. Physiologic basis for improved pulmonary function after lung volume reduction. Proceedings of the American Thoracic Society. 2008;**5**(4):416-420

[119] Zoumot Z, LoMauro A, Aliverti A, Nelson C, Ward S, Jordan S, et al. Lung volume reduction in emphysema improves chest wall asynchrony. Chest. 2015;**148**(1):185-195

[120] Johnson AN, Harkema JR, Nelson AJ, Dickinson JD, Kalil J, Duryee MJ, et al. MyD88 regulates a prolonged adaptation response to environmental dust exposure-induced lung disease. Respiratory Research. 2020;**21**:1-14

[121] Hummel JP, Mayse ML, Dimmer S, Johnson PJ. Physiologic and histopathologic effects of targeted lung denervation in an animal model. Journal of Applied Physiology. 2019;**126**(1):67-76

[122] Mayr AK, Valipour A. Modern Bronchoscopic treatment options for patients with chronic bronchitis. Journal of Clinical Medicine. 2023;**12**(5):1854

[123] Valipour A, Fernandez-Bussy S, Ing AJ, Steinfort DP, Snell GI, Williamson JP, et al. Bronchial rheoplasty for treatment of chronic bronchitis. Twelve-month results from a multicenter clinical trial. American Journal of Respiratory and Critical Care Medicine. 2020;**202**(5):681-689

[124] Leard LE, Holm AM, Valapour M, Glanville AR, Attawar S, Aversa M, et al. Consensus document for the selection of lung transplant candidates: An update from the International Society for Heart and Lung Transplantation. The Journal of Heart and Lung Transplantation. 2021;**40**(11):1349-1379

[125] Rampolla R. Lung transplantation: An overview of candidacy and outcomes. Ochsner Journal. 2014;**14**(4):641-648

[126] Verleden GM, Gottlieb J. Lung transplantation for COPD/pulmonary emphysema. European Respiratory Review. 2023;**32**(167):220116

[127] Snell G, Reed A, Stern M, Hadjiliadis D. The evolution of lung transplantation for cystic fibrosis: A 2017 update. Journal of Cystic Fibrosis. 2017;**16**(5):553-564

[128] Ramos KJ, Kapnadak SG, Bradford MC, Somayaji R, Morrell ED,

Pilewski JM, et al. Underweight patients with cystic fibrosis have acceptable survival following lung transplantation: A united network for organ sharing registry study. Chest. 2020;**157**(4):898-906

[129] van der Mark SC, Hoek RA, Hellemons ME. Developments in lung transplantation over the past decade. European Respiratory Review. 2020;**29**(157):190132

[130] Weill D. Lung transplantation: Indications and contraindications. Journal of Thoracic Disease. 2018;**10**(7):4574

[131] Lane CR, Tonelli AR. Lung transplantation in chronic obstructive pulmonary disease: Patient selection and special considerations. International Journal of Chronic Obstructive Pulmonary Disease. 2015;**10**:2137-2146

[132] Schaffer JM, Singh SK, Reitz BA, Zamanian RT, Mallidi HR. Single-vs double-lung transplantation in patients with chronic obstructive pulmonary disease and idiopathic pulmonary fibrosis since the implementation of lung allocation based on medical need. Journal of the American Medical Association. 2015;**313**(9):936-948

[133] Benvenuto LJ, Costa J, Piloni D, Aversa M, Anderson MR, Shah L, et al. Right single lung transplantation or double lung transplantation compared with left single lung transplantation in chronic obstructive pulmonary disease. The Journal of Heart and Lung Transplantation. 2020;**39**(9):870-877

[134] Sun Z, Li F, Zhou X, Chung KF, Wang W, Wang J. Stem cell therapies for chronic obstructive pulmonary disease: Current status of pre-clinical studies and clinical trials. Journal of Thoracic Disease. 2018;**10**(2):1084

[135] Kokturk N, Yıldırım F, Gülhan PY, Oh YM. Stem cell therapy in chronic obstructive pulmonary disease. How far is it to the clinic? American. Journal of Stem Cells. 2018;7(3):56

[136] Glassberg MK, Csete I, Simonet E, Elliot SJ. Stem cell therapy for COPD: Hope and exploitation. Chest. 2021;**160**(4):1271-1281

[137] Balkissoon R. Stem cell therapy for COPD: Where are we? Chronic Obstructive Pulmonary Diseases: Journal of the COPD Foundation. 2018;**5**(2):148

[138] Cruz FF, Rocco PRM. The potential of mesenchymal stem cell therapy for chronic lung disease. Expert Review of Respiratory Medicine. 2020;**14**(1):31-39

[139] Inamdar AC, Inamdar AA. Mesenchymal stem cell therapy in lung disorders: Pathogenesis of lung diseases and mechanism of action of mesenchymal stem cell. Experimental Lung Research. 2013;**39**(8):315-327

[140] Abbaszadeh H, Ghorbani F, Abbaspour-Aghdam S, Kamrani A, Valizadeh H, Nadiri M, et al. Chronic obstructive pulmonary disease and asthma: Mesenchymal stem cells and their extracellular vesicles as potential therapeutic tools. Stem Cell Research & Therapy. 2022;**13**(1):1-15

[141] Zarogoulidis P, Hohenforst-Schmidt W, Huang H, Sahpatzidou D, Freitag L, Sakkas L, et al. A gene therapy induced emphysema model and the protective role of stem cells. Diagnostic Pathology. 2014;**9**(1):1-7

[142] Jindal SK, Jindal A. Respiratory disorders: Contemporary issues in 2020. In: Biomedical Translational Research: From Disease Diagnosis to Treatment. Singapore: Springer Nature Singapore; 15 Jun 2022. pp. 181-194

[143] Thakur AK, Chellappan DK, Dua K, Mehta M, Satija S, Singh I. Patented therapeutic drug delivery strategies for targeting pulmonary diseases. Expert Opinion on Therapeutic Patents. 2020;**30**(5):375-387

[144] Bisserier M, Sun X, Fazal S, Turnbull I, Bonnet S, Hadri L. Novel insights into the therapeutic potential of lung-targeted gene transfer in the most common respiratory diseases. Cell. 2022;**11**:984 Note: MDPI stays neutral with regard to jurisdictional claims in published ...; 2022

[145] Calendine J, Batra S, Cherfils J, Said O, Nguyen V. Gene therapy avenues for chronic obstructive pulmonary disease. Berkeley Pharma Tech Journal of Medicine. 2022;**1**(2):58-80

[146] Katz MG, Fargnoli AS, Gubara SM, Fish K, Weber T, Bridges CR, et al. Targeted gene delivery through the respiratory system: Rationale for intratracheal gene transfer. Journal of Cardiovascular Development and Disease. 2019;**6**(1):8

[147] Stiles KM, Sondhi D, Kaminsky SM, De BP, Rosenberg JB, Crystal RG. Intrapleural gene therapy for alpha-1 antitrypsin deficiency-related lung disease. Chronic Obstructive Pulmonary Diseases: Journal of the COPD Foundation. 2018;**5**(4):244

[148] Karponi G, Zogas N, Domvri K, Zarogoulidis P, Trakada G, Roumeliotis S, et al. Prospects of gene therapy for pulmonary diseases: Progress and limitations. Medicinal Chemistry. 2017;**13**(4):308-318

[149] Kaufmann BK, Chiriaco M, Siler U, Finocchi A, Reichenbach J, Stein S, et al. Gene therapy for chronic granulomatous disease: Current status and future perspectives. Current Gene Therapy. 2014;**14**(6):447-460

[150] Harrell CR, Sadikot R, Pascual J, Fellabaum C, Jankovic MG, Jovicic N, et al. Mesenchymal stem cell-based therapy of inflammatory lung diseases: Current understanding and future perspectives. Stem Cells International. 2019;**2019**:14

[151] Domvri K, Zarogoulidis P, Porpodis K, Koffa M, Lambropoulou M, Kakolyris S, et al. Gene therapy in liver diseases: State-of-the-art and future perspectives. Current Gene Therapy. 2012;**12**(6):463-483